D0725206

F

Pe

The cover design shows the Basket of Wooden Objects described on page 87, the Feely Fish (page 90), the Chopping Board Jigsaw (page 97) and the Noughts and Crosses game from page 103. The background is from the Large Draughts Board described on page 104.

FUN AND GAMES
Practical Leisure Ideas for People with Profound Disabilities

JUDY DENZILOE

Illustrated by Gillian Hunter

Foreword by
Roy McConkey

Director of Training and Research,
St Aidan's, Melrose

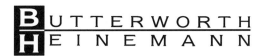

BUTTERWORTH
HEINEMANN

Butterworth-Heinemann Ltd
Linacre House, Jordan Hill, Oxford OX2 8DP

℞ A member of the Reed Elsevier plc group

OXFORD LONDON BOSTON
MUNICH NEW DELHI SINGAPORE SYDNEY
TOKYO TORONTO WELLINGTON

First published 1994
Reprinted 1995

British Library Cataloguing in Publication Data
Denziloe, Judy
  Fun and Games: Practical leisure ideas
  for people with profound disabilities
  I. Title
  790.1

ISBN 0 7506 0571 5

Library of Congress Cataloguing in Publication Data
Denziloe, Judy
  Fun and games: practical leisure ideas for people with profound
  disabilities/Judy Denziloe; illustrated by Gillian Hunter;
  foreword by Roy McConkey.
  p. cm.
  Includes bibliographical references and index.
  ISBN 0 7506 0571 5
  1. Recreation therapy. 2. Handicapped – Recreation. I. Title.
  [DNLM: 1. Disabled. 2. Play and Playthings.   WB 320 D417f 1994]
  RM736.7.D46
  615.8'5153 – dc20   93-36031
                                                                  CIP

Typeset by TecSet Ltd, Wallington, Surrey
Printed and bound in Great Britain by The Bath Press, Avon

Contents

Contents

Foreword

Why do humans play? The popular answer – 'for the fun of it' – is only partly true. You need only recall the seriousness with which children get absorbed in their play and the upsets which can arise, to realize that play can be hard work! The 'excess energy' theory – that the human mind and body need to be fully occupied – is equally incomplete. Play is often most therapeutic when we are tired and care-worn. And play must be more than a pass-time. How else do you explain the terrific diversity, not to say complexity of the many play activities which humans have invented?

Judy Denziloe has a clear belief in the purpose of play. 'It is essential', she writes, for human 'physical, mental, emotional, social and spiritual development' (p. 5). Many would agree with her.

It is doubly ironic then that the very people in our society whose development is most jeopardized – those with profound disabilities – are the very ones most likely to be deprived of opportunities to play or to engage in productive leisure pursuits. Some would say the reasons are obvious. Disability is a serious business. These people need treatment and therapy not fun and games. And anyway such 'patients' are incapable of playing; they are content to lie doing nothing.

Fortunately the accepted wisdom of years past has given way to new insights. Christopher Nolan, the Irish writer with such profound disabilities that he is totally dependent on others, recalls in his autobiography, a family holiday when he was taken swimming in the 'billowing' Atlantic ocean. 'He glowed with pleasure as he skimmed along, for he felt totally relaxed and safe in their hands and through their efforts he sampled the joys of the able-bodied' (Nolan, p. 104). As Christopher's story illustrates and this book amply demonstrates, it is the inventiveness and determination of mature players which enables them to join in the game.

On these pages is the most complete collection of ideas for activities and playthings I have come across. Better still, most of them have been tried and tested through Judy's work with children and adults with profound disabilities in home, hospital and community settings. Many are embarrassingly simple to put into practice: an indictment to the sceptics who claim they lack time or money. Nor has the cry – 'we have tried everything and nothing has worked' – any credibility when faced with the evidence presented here.

Ultimately though, changes in practice come from changed attitudes. Do we really believe that play and leisure are essential to human well-being and secondly that everyone, no matter how profound their disability needs to experience fun and games? One final word of advice: why not begin by joining in the fun and games using the ideas presented here and see what effect that has on your attitudes. As they say, seeing is believing!

Roy McConkey

Nolan, C. (1987) *Under the Eye of the Clock*, London: Pan Books

Acknowledgements

It is just over twenty years since I decided that I didn't want to be a scientist and started working in the field of play and leisure. Since then many people — both disabled and non-disabled — have influenced, inspired and supported me and I am grateful to all of them. They are, as the saying goes, too numerous to mention but I hope they know who they are and how much I value the contact we have, or had in the past.

I would like to thank all the people who have shared ideas with me, both in the past and specifically for inclusion in this book. Also the authors who gave permission for their designs, which have been published elsewhere, to be included here.

Special thanks are due to my mother, who spotted the original job advertisement which got me involved in this area of work, and who has always given me so much encouragement.

Thanks also to my colleagues in Planet who have kept the project going during my writing weeks, and who have been too polite to comment when my mind has obviously been full of the book at other times!

Love and gratitude to my husband, Phil, who has put up with so much over the years. We met through a 'Making toys' workshop so perhaps he knew what he was letting himself in for, but I'm sure he wasn't prepared for the junk materials and half-finished projects cluttering the house or the favours asked (he has access to wonderful woodworking machines!).

I would like to thank Gillian Hunter for her lovely illustrations which accompany instructions for making equipment — I am sure they will help the reader to make sense of my written descriptions!

Introduction

All About Me

In 1972 I graduated with a science degree with very little idea of what I wanted to do with my life, apart from the conviction that I did not want to be a scientist! By chance, my local health authority was looking for a graduate to start two of the first toy libraries in long-stay hospitals and thus began nine very happy years running a toy library in a comprehensive children's hospital and a leisure equipment library in a hospital for adults with learning disabilities.

I particularly enjoyed my work with adults, and the challenge of finding suitable equipment. 'Normalization' and 'age appropriateness' were unheard of, but I had firm views on play and leisure and the types of equipment and materials I felt comfortable with. Very little commercial leisure equipment was being designed for this client group, some items in the educational catalogues were suitable, but for most situations the answer was 'do it yourself'. Fortunately I had always enjoyed making things, both in fabric and in wood, and the obvious leisure needs sparked off plenty of ideas. Buying a piece of equipment which proves popular is satisfying, but nothing beats the feeling when you make something that's a success!

In 1981 I went to work for the Toy Libraries Association (now Play Matters/The National Association of Toy and Leisure Libraries), initially with responsibility for the work of ACTIVE and equipment for people with disabilities, and later for training and publications as well. Four years later I was employed by Save the Children to manage Playtrac, a mobile training resource on play and leisure for people with learning disabilities.

Following the successful handover of Playtrac to the North West Thames Regional Health Authority in 1988, I remained with Save the Children to develop a new project of which I am now the manager. Planet is a national information resource on play, leisure and recreation for children, young people and adults with disabilities. Thus leisure for adults, and particularly those with profound disabilities, remains a focus of my work and a special interest.

1

This Book

When Butterworth-Heinemann approached me to write a book about leisure for adults with profound disabilities, my first reaction was 'I can't write a book' and my second was that visitors to Planet seem to find my ideas useful so perhaps it was time they were put down on paper. It was important to me that Butterworth-Heinemann wanted a practical book, to continue the series started by Roma Lear's excellent books 'Play Helps' and 'More Play Helps' — partly because that is the only type of book I would want to write, but also because I would be in such wonderful company. Roma has been a friend and an inspiration for most of my working life and my first move, when I started work on 'Fun and Games' was to ask Roma's permission to include a few of her designs in my book. These are pieces of equipment which are, in my opinion, suitable for adults, but people working in adult services are unlikely to find them because they are in books about children's play.

I also wrote to several journals, some aimed at professionals and others for parents, to ask people to submit ideas for inclusion in the book. The response was very disappointing. I think there are several possible reasons for this — people are too busy to put pen to paper, or they think their ideas aren't very good or are so simple that everyone else will have thought of them. Sadly, I suspect the other reason is that, for many people with profound disabilities, leisure opportunities are very restricted and unexciting.

I contacted about thirty leisure libraries which specialize in lending equipment to adults. Of those who replied, most said that they did not cater for people with profound disabilities (although they would do so if asked) and those that did mainly stocked musical instruments, computers and switch-operated items.

I would like to thank those people whose ideas do appear in this book — the few who responded to my letters in the journals and those who were willing to share ideas when they visited Planet, or when I met them during my travels round the country. Also the friends and colleagues who willingly gave permission for their designs, which had been published elsewhere, to appear in 'Fun and Games'. All the books they come from are very popular in Planet's library and I hope readers will be motivated to seek them out for further information and ideas.

Originality

It is always difficult to be 100 per cent confident about the originality of a design — different people, facing similar problems or challenges, are quite likely to come up with similar solutions. The designs which are credited to me are ones which I developed during the 1970s in my leisure equipment library. The designs which have been given to me by other people have been accepted in good faith as their own. Ideas which are not attributed are those which I have gathered together over the years.

Safety

The aim of this book is to share leisure ideas and to enable you to make pieces of equipment. Where the full instructions have been given, great care has been taken to make them as clear and accurate as possible. However, neither I nor the publishers have any control over the skills of the people who may be making the equipment and we cannot accept responsibility for the results. Please think carefully before tackling a project — have you got the necessary skills, do you need to ask someone with more experience to show you how to use the tools ? Please read chapter 2, and in particular the section on Safety, before you begin any project.

Commercial Equipment

Including commercial equipment in a book like this inevitably causes problems, as products cease to be available very quickly. However, information on commercial equipment only forms a small part of the book and I think it is important to highlight successful items. Also, if good designs go out of production then they should be rescued by other manufacturers or give inspiration for DIY ideas.

Terminology

I look at articles and leaflets I wrote years ago and wince at the language used! I don't think my values or the respect I have for people needed to change very much, but my feelings about the terminology I am comfortable with certainly have changed.

Trying to clarify the intended audience for this book inevitably involves labelling people, but I have tried to keep this to a minimum. The ideas and equipment in this book are divided up by how they can be used and what the outcomes might be, not by the type of person who could take part.

'Fun and Games' is concerned with practical leisure ideas for people with a profound learning disability or multiple disabilities, but that is only a general guide to what you will find in its pages. You know your son or daughter, or the people you work with — their abilities, likes and dislikes. I hope there are some ideas here that will be enjoyed by them — and by you!

I hope that the book will be of use to parents and other family members, friends, staff and volunteers — anyone who is interested in the leisure needs of people with profound disabilities. I have used the term 'enabler' for anyone who may be introducing these leisure ideas. For most of the time, the words 'person' or 'people' are all that are needed to describe those who may benefit from the ideas. Where another word is needed, I have used 'client' as this seems to be a generally accepted term for people who find themselves passing their time in various informal and formal settings.

3

Another aspect of terminology is what we should call the pieces of equipment described in the book. Using the word 'toy' would alienate many readers who believe, quite rightly, that adults with disabilities should not be treated as children. We talk about 'executive toys' and if someone has a new car, computer or mobile phone we often call it the 'new toy' but we seem to have a real problem with what to call the objects used by people with profound disabilities for leisure and pleasure.

In this book you will find 'equipment', 'object', 'item' or the name of the design used to describe leisure materials. This can become very cumbersome and may be irritating to the reader — perhaps it will serve as a useful reminder that it is our hang-ups about the words 'play' and 'toys' in association with the word 'adult' which makes this necessary.

The issue of whether adults play is explored in the next chapter.

. . . And Finally

It is said that everyone has one book in them — this is mine. It gathers together ideas which I have used or seen used over the last twenty years. I hope it will be a useful contribution to the debate about leisure for people with profound disabilities but, above all, I hope that its contribution will be a practical one and that the ideas for activities and equipment will help to increase leisure opportunities for this section of the community.

1

Play and Leisure

What is Play?

Play is a basic human activity. It is essential for a child's physical, mental, emotional, social and spiritual development. It needs few external rewards, the satisfaction and enjoyment are in the **process** and very rarely in the **end-product**, if indeed there is one.

Play is a freely chosen, spontaneous activity. The same activity may be done in various contexts — play, education, work — but the play activity can be recognized by the intention behind the activity and the way in which it is performed. There are various verbal and non-verbal signals which convey the message 'I am playing', such as smiling and laughter, or the 'play face' in monkeys — in a play fight, it is essential that both sides know that it is not the real thing, otherwise there are problems!

There are many contradictions in play. It is usually considered to be an activity which is free from the constraints of real life and not governed by reality. Yet in play the child practises skills which she will need in life and acts out roles and situations. Play has its own rules and goals. So does real life, but they are different. It is the **context** which distinguishes play and real life — within play the child's actions are not linked to real goals and consequences.

Caillois (1961) listed the formal characteristics of play:

- **free** — play is not obligatory, if it were then it would lose its attractive and joyous qualities;
- **separate** — contained within limits of space and time, defined and fixed in advance;
- **uncertain** — neither the course nor the result of play are known beforehand, it develops according to the player's initiative;
- **unproductive** — no goods or wealth are created, the situation is the same at the end as at the beginning;
- **governed by rules** — which are established in the play situation and temporarily suspend rules in the external world;
- **make believe** — a special awareness of a different reality, or an unreality, from real life.

Do Adults Play?

'Play may sound a strange word when talking about adults. But adults do, or can, play. Play is whenever someone explores something to discover more about it or himself **for the enjoyment of it all**' (Blackburn, undated). That view was expressed in a booklet published in the early 1970s. Between then and now, very little has been written about adult play although there are one or two fragments of comment and research in amongst all the academic papers on play.

'Adults play when they have nothing better to do; in fact a philosopher once described adult play as "useless in the eyes of the beholder". But that is not to say it has no function at all; it is probably essential as a means of relaxation' (Einon, 1985). How can an author who believes strongly in the importance and creativity of children's play be so dismissive of the adult activity?

'The poet has it that man is never more human than when he plays. But what must he do and be, and in what context, to be both adult and playful: must he do something in which he feels again as if he were a playing child, or a youth in a game? Must he step outside of his most serious and most fateful concerns? Or must he transcend his everyday condition and be "beside himself" in fantasy, ecstasy or "togetherness"? . . . The adult once was a child and a youth. He will never be either again: but neither will he ever be without the heritage of those former states. In fact, I would postulate that, in order to be truly adult, he must on each level renew some of the playfulness of childhood and some of the sportiveness of the young' (Erikson, 1976).

Many studies have shown a link between adult playfulness and creativity, imagination, improvisation and spontaneity. In an interview in 1992, when he was 70 years old, Michael Bentine explained why he thought it was a good idea for adults to play with toys: 'If you want to shape up your creativity the best thing to do is use a focus, and the two best foci are books and toys'.

Young animals play to practise hunting and fighting skills, and for their social development, but adult animals also play. Polecats, dogs, wolves, otters and badgers have all been observed to play, not to practise skills or as sexual behaviour but simply because they are feeling joyful, carefree, or because the sun is shining. This extract comes from an American article on comparative behaviour in Cetaceans; I do not know the exact reference, but it is such a beautiful quotation that it must be included here: 'Extreme playfulness and humour are conspicuous in dolphins and may be found in whales also, although they are harder to observe. Despite its low status in puritanical value systems, play is a hallmark of intelligence and is indispensable for creativity and flexibility. Its marked development in Cetaceans makes it likely that they will frolic with their minds as much as with their bodies'.

Attitudes towards play are strongly influenced by cultural values. In Western society young children and old people are allowed to play more and the playfulness of creative and artistic people is tolerated. The rest of us are expected to work and only play at certain times in clearly defined situations. The presence of young children or domestic pets is often used as an excuse to play. Other cultures, and other periods of Western history have a very different — and, I believe, a much healthier — attitude towards play, with families and communities playing together.

Our traditional distinction between work (valuable) and play (a waste of time) is often blamed on the 'Protestant work ethic', but this is not accurate. Certainly the 17th- and 18th-century Puritans and Quakers disapproved of gambling, unseemly behaviour in dancing, and so on, but they believed that play had a function as a counterbalance to work. However, because of their obsession with time (which should be used to serve God) they believed that play and recreation should not occupy an excessive amount of time.

Our industrial society tends to compartmentalize work and leisure, but play does not fit into this scheme because play can happen anytime, any place. Play can happen during work, to relieve the boredom and to build social relationships. Various studies have identified play opportunities in work situations:

1. 'mucking about' type of horseplay, when out of sight of supervisors and managers;
2. practical jokes, such as sending new apprentices to the stores for non-existent tools;
3. day dreaming and fantasy 'mind games', while hands and eyes are absorbed in routine tasks;
4. developing sign language to communicate in noisy environments
5. taking pride in doing a job well, and competing to see who is the most skilful, have many similarities to play;
6. putting on work clothing (a uniform or safety clothing, for example) is putting on a role, like an actor or player.

Many researchers equate adult play with sports and games, but I believe there are important differences. Initially a sporting activity may show some of the features of play — voluntary involvement, fun, lack of external rewards — but as it is played at higher levels, the emphasis is on competition, strict rules and success.

In his study of spontaneous adult play, Bowman (1978) identifies two consistencies in play:

1. people are able to recognize and achieve a sense of play in their everyday interactions;
2. play signals are clearly understood within and between species.

He defines spontaneous adult play as occasions where playfulness emerges during interaction and participants actively negotiate new rules and create new games (not formally organized games and sports). An example is ball play. There are formalized games, such as football or cricket, but spontaneous play could include kicking the ball about, throwing it in the air or at each other, 'piggy in the middle'. The play is less systematic and more open-ended; it is often co-operative rather than competitive.

7

In spontaneous play one action leads to another, changing the nature of the play. The players need sensitivity to pick up the cues so that the activity changes and develops as the players want it to. Adult play may be signalled by explicit verbal statements or questions, such as 'Let's just play' or 'Are we going to keep score or are we just going to play?', or by non-verbal cues such as facial expressions, exaggerated or repeated movements.

Adult play is very fragile — it stops if the action gets too rough, if spectators appear to be annoyed or disapproving, or if the players start to analyse what they are doing. The activities are often, but not always, triggered by a childhood memory: rolling down a grassy slope, throwing autumn leaves over each other or up in the air, play fighting and wrestling, water fights, playing with bubbles.

Bowman suggests that adult play has many features in common with children's play:

1. the players are completely engrossed in the process and developing the activity;
2. the meaning and significance of what they are doing is not analysed;
3. the play is improvisational, co-operative and fun;
4. it needs an accepting and supportive environment.

In his study of the development of play, Cohen (1987) devotes a chapter to adults. He identifies four areas of adult play:

1. participation in sports, especially dangerous ones;
2. computer and fantasy games;
3. adult toys;
4. therapy games.

He suggests that people with routine or mundane jobs are particularly drawn to high risk sports, as they seek the thrills which are missing from their lives. But play should be safe, stress-free and separate from reality. The possible consequences in high risk sports — injury or death — are all too real, so can we call this play?

Fantasy games are often warlike and aggressive. The suppliers claim that they encourage imagination, but this is not true — there are only certain things you can do in the game and the possible actions and outcomes are controlled by the imagination of the creator, not the player. Is this play?

There are various types of adult toys. Some people will always want the latest gadget — a new hi-fi with more knobs and flashing lights, for example. Others buy useless objects to demonstrate how wealthy they are. Shops and catalogues highlight 'presents for the person who has everything'. Soft toys are purchased by, and for, adults. Stress dolls (soft dolls with limbs attached by Velcro, so that they can be pulled apart) and stress heads (filled with gel, which can be squeezed and poked) encourage a healthy release of tension, but in an unpleasant way because the objects resemble people.

Executive toys are popular, but people usually feel more comfortable with them if they can be claimed to demonstrate a scientific principle (like

Newton's Cradle) or to be a sculpture (like Pin Sculpture or magnetic constructions). As Cohen says 'the things that sell as toys for adults still reflect our unease about playing as grown ups'. Adults buy toys but they rarely know how to play with them; indeed, many of them are for display rather than play.

Many types of 'therapy games' — encounter groups, assertiveness training, complementary therapies (holistic massage, aromatherapy, etc.) resemble play. People choose to attend the group or activity in their free time, there is a clear structure to the activities and a time limit. The group operates outside real life. Role playing has many obvious links with play and can be used to explore feelings, try out other people's roles, in job training, in fantasy, or as therapy. Cohen suggests that the increasing popularity of role playing is blurring the traditional distinctions between work and play and that stressed executives are becoming involved in many activities which bear at least a superficial resemblance to play. 'Adults may feel inhibited by the thought that they are doing something that only children do and so bring into their "play" many of the stresses of real life. Americans tend to admire men and women who work *hard* and play *hard*. Perhaps we need to convince ourselves that it is more than possible to play soft, to play playfully or, even, to work playfully. . . . We ought to develop our play from womb to tomb. . . . There is no way of proving it but it is plausible, at least, that a world in which adults felt freer to play would be a happier and less dangerous one'.

What is Leisure?

Play is an innate need, leisure is an artificial creation. Leisure became an increasingly important part of people's lives as society became more industrialized; it was viewed as the opposite of work. This is not a helpful way of describing leisure — when work is seen as valuable, the implication is that leisure is not. We should instead regard leisure as an essential component in everyone's life alongside work (possibly), chores and other responsibilities. In our post-industrial society, with increasing unemployment and other changes in work patterns, it is essential to give leisure the status it deserves so that people who have large amounts of leisure time are also valued.

We may use leisure time for relaxation, stimulation, developing new skills, building our social networks or releasing our creativity. Leisure can be viewed in various ways:

1. as **activity** — some activities involve planning, use of facilities or equipment and the involvement of other people. Others are much more spontaneous;
2. as **time** — leisure takes place in 'non-obligated time' in other words, those occasions when we are free of responsibilities and the demands of others;
3. as **state of mind** — when we feel free to choose our activity to please ourselves, without external pressures or rewards.

The terms 'leisure', 'recreation' and 'sport' are used interchangeably by many people, but I believe there are important differences. Recreation is taking part in physical activities which produce a feeling of well-being and revitalization. Sports are those activities which are competitive, controlled by strict rules, records and traditions and in which the outcome is mainly determined by physical skill. Some activities, e.g. cycling or swimming, can be recreation or sport but the context is different.

There are many influences on our choice of leisure activities:

- Class, culture, social background, lifestyle
- Gender
- Money
- Transport
- Availability of facilities
- Personality (preference for solitary or group activities, for example)
- Opportunities available in childhood
- Influence of family and friends
- Expectations, attitudes and values
- Self-confidence
- Abilities — our perceptions of our own abilities

All these can affect the leisure of people with disabilities but another major factor is enablers' perceptions of people's abilities which often restrict the information and choices available to them.

Lack of choice and powerlessness to take control is one of the most disabling features of people's lives. Dattilo and Rusch (1985) studied the effect of choice on leisure participation and suggested that:

1. people with disabilities are not provided with sufficient opportunities to make leisure choices, especially if they have severe disabilities;
2. continuous involvement in situations which fail to provide opportunities for choice may result in feelings of helplessness;
3. learned helplessness may result in withdrawal, which compounds the individual's disability;
4. people who have learned that their actions have no effect on the environment may cease to do anything.

Edgerton (1967), in a study of people with learning disabilities living in the community, wrote 'The use of leisure time indicates better than anything else the richness or impoverishment of their lives.' Tyne (1978) found a tendency towards passive and home-based activities (such as watching television) among residents of a group home and commented that they 'appeared to lead curiously unstimulating lives'.

Atkinson (1985) found some improvement in the number of activities which were being enjoyed by people who had moved from hospital into the community, but very few of the activities were ones which would encourage social integration. She found four main problems:

1. giving up pursuits (usually due to lack of money or poor health);
2. getting stuck — not knowing how to extend a hobby, by joining a local club for instance;
3. the threshold — an activity may take the person into the community as a spectator, but not as a participant;
4. few people join in participatory activities (e.g. keep fit, sports, evening classes) which ensure contact with other people but also involve the risk of failure, of not being able to do the activity.

People with profound disabilities are likely to face even more barriers to participation in the leisure life of the community. Many leisure facilities are much more accessible now, but do they offer appropriate activities? What would be the reaction if adults with profound disabilities wanted to use the soft play area and ballpool in a leisure centre, when non-disabled adults are not expected or allowed to? Will we see the day when multisensory environments are installed in leisure centres, for everyone's use?

Age-appropriateness

The concept of age-appropriateness is an important one, but the judgements which have to be made are very subjective — what is acceptable to one enabler, another will consider childish. It is a concept which was developed by authoritative people and is implemented by enablers — it is unlikely that the person with profound disabilities has much contribution to the debate.

The picture of an adult using a child's toy may be degrading and is likely to affect, either consciously or subconsciously, the way we relate to that person. More important, the toy is unlikely to be suitable in terms of size, complexity and the life experiences it reflects.

Normalization, from whence came the concept of age-appropriateness, is often quoted as the reason for not allowing play. However, Smith (1985) wrote 'Normalisation should not be used as an excuse for witholding play and recreational facilities from adults with mental handicap as in reality there is no conflict except for those who misinterpret, or do not understand, the principles.'

Surely the question is 'Do we value play and leisure in our own lives?' If so, then these opportunities should be available to everyone.

Age-appropriateness is only one aspect to be considered when selecting or designing equipment. It is essential that the person's skill level, experiences and interests are taken into account, as well as their age.

It is ironic that the example most frequently used to illustrate the 'problem' of age-appropriateness — finding simple jigsaws with suitable pictures — is the easiest to solve. Some specialist companies supply adult jigsaws and it is easy to make your own (see chapter 7). Other aspects of the issue are not so simple. Ask a group of enablers if they are happy to use a child's plastic stacking ring toy with an adult and they are likely to reply 'No'. Ask if they would be happy if the stacking toy was made of wood with beautifully carved and stained rings and several will probably say 'Yes'. In

11

my opinion, they are missing the point. Substituting one item for another is purely cosmetic — it is no more appropriate for an adult to be sitting at a table stacking wooden rings than it would be if they were plastic. It is the activity which is inappropriate, not just the equipment. If the person needs to learn the skill involved, then this can be done in a teaching session, with whichever stacking toy the person prefers and finds easier to use, as a step towards using the skill in everyday situations.

Many of today's adults with disabilities were children at a time when they were considered ineducable (pre-1971); they have experienced years of deprivation and restricted opportunities. The introduction of new activities may be met with resistance at first. The physical and mental effort required can be very tiring; new experiences may be frightening and the response to any new sensation may be withdrawal.

In recent years, many children and young people with profound disabilities have experienced a much wider range of activities — the sensory curriculum, multisensory environments, soft play areas, ball pools, hydrotherapy, Soundbeam, outdoor adventure, to name a few. As adults they will have much higher expectations, both for their daytime occupation and in their leisure activities — it is up to us to meet this challenge.

In 1984 I wrote 'There is a danger that preconceived ideas about play and a desire to embrace new policies will lead those who care for people with disabilities to deny some of their most basic rights — the right to learn and practise new skills, to face challenges and solve problems and to seek relaxation, emotional fulfilment and social interaction through enjoyable activities'. I see no reason to change my view — if we acknowledge our own need for both leisure *and* play in our lives then we will be better able to offer a range of appropriate activities and support people in the choices they make.

References

Atkinson, D. (1985), *With Time to Spare: the Leisure Pursuits of People with Mental Handicaps*, Mental Handicap, 13 Dec 1985.

Blackburn, D. (undated), *Play for Mentally Handicapped Adults*, Toy Libraries Association.

Bowman, John R., (1978), 'The organization of spontaneous adult social play', In *Play: Anthropological Perspectives*, Michael A. Salter (ed.), Leisure Press N.Y.

Caillois, R., (1961), *Man, Play and Games* (M. Barash, trans.), Free Press.

Cohen, D., (1987), *The Development of Play*, Croom Helm.

Dattilo, J. and Rusch, F.R., (1985), *Effects of Choice on Leisure Participation for Persons with Severe Handicaps*, J.Assoc. for Persons with Severe Handicaps, 10(4), 1985.

Edgerton, R.B., (1967), *The Cloak of Competence*, Berkley: Univ. California Press.

Einon, D., (1985), *Creative Play: Play with a Purpose from Birth to Ten Years*, Penguin.

Erikson, Eric H. (1976), 'Play and actuality, In *Play: Its Role in Development and Evolution*', J.S. Bruner, A. Jolly and K. Sylva (eds), Penguin.

Smith, S., (1985), *Normalisation, Play and Recreation*, The Spastics Society.

Tyne, A., (1978), *Looking at Life in a Hospital, Hostel, Home or Unit*, CMH, London.

2

Doing It Yourself – or Getting Someone to Do It For You!

Why Make Equipment ?

There are several reasons why you may choose to make play and leisure equipment:

1. appropriate equipment is not available commercially;
2. you can make the piece of equipment to meet the needs of the person who will use it;
3. you can reflect the person's interests, experiences and culture in the design and decoration of the item;
4. the finished product will almost certainly be cheaper than a commercial item;
5. the pleasure and satisfaction of working with your hands and creating something.

It is important to distinguish between making an item which is not available commercially, or which is similar to a commercial item but more suitable for the person, and making an exact copy of an item which you could have bought from a shop or catalogue. It is wrong to make a copy and rarely very successful.

I remember visiting a unit some years ago and being shown a copy of a large wall cogboard which had been made by a local workshop. At the time the cogboard, a beautiful piece of equipment with sixteen large cogs which interlock and rotate, must have been selling for about £200. I tried to turn the cogs on the copy and found that they did not fit together properly, so they would not rotate smoothly. 'It doesn't work very well' said the manager of the unit, 'but it only cost us £30 for materials'.

What a waste of everyone's time! If the manager had talked to some local charities they would probably have been pleased to donate the equipment. The workshop trainees could have concentrated on making items which were within their capabilities. The clients in the unit would have been spared the

13

frustration of trying to use a piece of equipment which failed to respond correctly.

Ideas

Where do the ideas come from when you decide to make a piece of equipment? In many cases you will look at the person and know what she needs, all you have to do is decide how to make it. Sometimes an illustration in a catalogue will spark off an idea — 'that would be great if only if it was bigger, brighter and made a noise', for example.

There are books (including this one!) which give instructions for making equipment. You may want to follow the directions exactly, or modify them to meet your needs and the materials you have available. ACTIVE (see chapter 10) publishes a series of worksheets which include some excellent designs for leisure equipment.

Tools Needed

Obviously what tools you use will depend on the piece of equipment you have chosen to make, but the lists below give some indication of the range of tools you may need.

Woodwork

The most important item is a suitable surface to work on. A Workmate is ideal because it is stable and it is easy to position pieces of wood to work on them. A workbench is fine, otherwise a sturdy, solid table will do — but it will need protecting from damage.

A bench hook will also prove useful. You can buy these, but they are very easy to make. You will need a piece of blockboard approximately 20 cm × 30 cm and two pieces of softwood 4 cm square and 15 cm long. Glue and screw the softwood in position, as shown in the diagram. If you are left handed, the gap should be on the left side. The bench hook is used for sawing pieces of dowel or soft wood — as you hold the wood against the rest, you are pressing the bench hook against the workbench so that everything is held firmly while you saw.

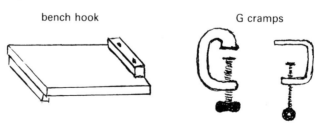

bench hook   G cramps

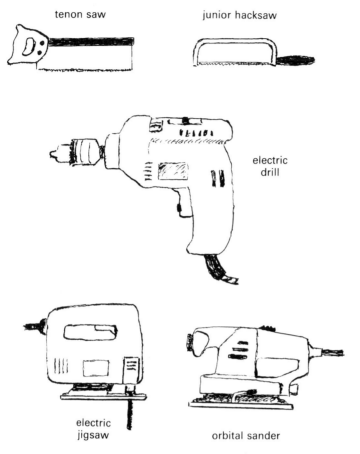

tenon saw   junior hacksaw

electric
drill

electric
jigsaw

orbital sander

If you have access to power tools — an electric drill, jigsaw, sander and planer — and someone to teach you how to use them, they will make your job a lot easier and quicker. Treated with respect and used under supervision, power tools can enable even novice woodworkers to achieve results they can be proud of. Use cordless tools (e.g. drill) when possible.

The other tools you will need are:

- Hammer
- Screwdrivers — various sizes, for slotted screws and for crosspoint
- Hand drill (even if you have an electric drill, a hand drill is useful for various jobs, such as making small starter holes for screws)
- Set of twist drills, flat woodbits and countersink drill
- Tenon saw
- Junior hacksaw
- G cramps (to clamp wood down while you work on it)
- Surform, files and sandpaper for smoothing wood
- Paintbrushes, various sizes, to apply paint and varnish

One piece of kitchen equipment I find very useful is a wire cooling tray (for baking cakes). Pieces of wood (e.g. jigsaw pieces) which have been painted or

15

varnished can stick to the newpaper they have been placed on to dry. Place them on the wire tray (standing on some newspaper, in case of drips) and any 'runs' won't matter.

You will also need some scrap pieces of wood. Large pieces are needed to go under your wood when you are drilling holes; this helps to stop the underside of the wood breaking away as the drill goes through, and also protects the surface you are resting on. Small scraps of plywood are useful when you are clamping wood down — place them between the wood and the G cramp to prevent it marking the wood as you tighten the screw.

Sewing

A reliable sewing machine which can do zig-zag stitching really is a must. You will also need sharp scissors in various sizes. (I prefer to keep my needlework scissors purely for that purpose, so that their blades are not sticky with Sellotape, blunted by paper, or damaged in any way.)

As well as ordinary sewing needles, you will need some with large eyes for use with the thicker threads which are sometimes needed for strength.

Use glass-headed pins, which show up better in the fabric. Always count the number of pins you have used and make sure that you remove the same number.

Working with Paper, Card and Textures

You will need sharp scissors, and a craft knife or scalpel. (You can buy disposable ones with plastic handles or metal scalpels which you can fit with replacement blades.) Cutting card accurately or trimming textures stuck on wooden shapes is much easier with a knife than with scissors. Use a metal rule to guide the knife for cutting straight lines. If you use a plastic ruler, the sharp knife may start to shave off bits of plastic and your line will not be straight! If you find that the rule slips as you are cutting, stick it to the card with two tiny blobs of Blutac.

When cutting with a craft knife you can rest your work on a piece of scrap plywood, but the blade will be blunted very quickly. You could use a proper cutting board, from a graphic supplies shop, but they are expensive. This is where another piece of kitchen equipment comes in useful — a plastic chopping board. It is an ideal surface to work on and will not blunt your knife.

Materials

For wooden equipment you will need:

1. Plywood — made up of thin sheets of wood laminated together and available in various thicknesses. Choose good quality wood, avoid pieces which are split, warped, or where the layers are separating.

2. Blockboard — rectangular strips of softwood glued side by side and sandwiched between thin veneers of wood. It is cheaper than plywood and useful for chunky jigsaws and bases for pieces of equipment. Avoid chipboard (wood chips stuck together with glue, usually faced with a wood veneer) — the cut edges may crumble away and you will need special chipboard screws.
3. Hardboard — very little strength; useful for jigsaw trays and backing inset boards and used for some of the items in this book. Pegboard is hardboard with rows of holes drilled in it.
4. Dowel and square or rectangular section softwood — either pine or ramin (slightly harder), available in various sizes.

You can, of course, use hardwoods but they are very expensive and more difficult to work with — probably best left to skilled craftspeople.

Most wood mills and timber yards sell offcuts of wood at very reasonable prices. In many cases you can let the size of the offcut dictate the size of the object but if you want a particular sized square or rectangle, it may be worth asking the staff at the wood mill to cut it accurately for you on their bandsaw (probably for a small charge) if you are not used to handling a saw.

Finishes for wood — once you have made your wooden object, the surface will need sealing in some way to protect it and to enable you to keep it clean. Make sure that the surface of the wood is smooth and dry and brush off any loose sawdust. You can leave the wood plain (i.e. uncoloured) and apply varnish. This brings out the grain of the wood and can look very attractive, but I sometimes wonder if it appeals more to us than to the people who are going to use the equipment!

You may prefer to colour the wood. Further details of coloured finishes are given in the section on Safety (below). Most of these finishes will require varnish on top to make them waterproof and hardwearing.

When varnishing, it is better to apply several thin coats than a few thick ones. Allow each coat to dry completely before applying the next. If you leave some varnish on the bristles and wrap them tightly in a plastic bag, excluding as much air as possible, the brush will stay soft while each coat dries and you won't have to clean it until you have finished. Choose a varnish with a matt or silk finish, rather than a high gloss one which could cause a dazzling glare for people with a visual impairment.

For other projects you will need:

● Fabric, especially interesting textures like velvet, towelling, synthetic fur, etc.
● Polyester stuffing or old tights cut up into small pieces, for stuffing fabric shapes; polyester wadding for padding mats.
● Foam plastic (sold in some upholstery shops for replacement cushions, or look in Yellow Pages under Foam Products — Plastic).
● Scraps of ribbon, tape, upholstery trimmings (fringes, bobbles, etc.)
● Buttons, beads, sequins.
● Nylon rope, piping cord, plastic tubing.

- Paper, card, cellophane, acetate, foil.
- Velcro — the 'hook and loop' fastener, one of the best inventions ever. You will probably need three types: the one you sew onto fabric, stick'n'sew (one half self-adhesive, the other to sew on) and the one where both sides are self-adhesive.
- Sellotape or masking tape — for temporarily anchoring things down. For more permanent use (e.g. reinforcing cardboard storage boxes or repairing books) use Scotch Magic Tape, which won't dry out or go sticky like Sellotape does.
- PVC tape (sold as insulating tape) — strong, sticks well, available in a range of colours.
- Fablon — available in various plain colours, also a textured green 'baize'.
- Self adhesive clear plastic (e.g. Transpaseal) — this can be bought in small quantities from stationers. It is much more economic to order a large roll from an office stationers or the educational catalogues. Used for covering pictures, etc. to protect them.
- Adhesives — you will need a range, for different purposes:
    Wood glue (e.g. Evostick)
    Copydex (for fabrics)
    General purpose adhesive (e.g. Bostik, UHU)
    Araldite
    Spray mount (available from stationers and graphics supplies shops, used for mounting pictures or photographs on card)
    PVA glue (sold for school use, excellent glue for sticking paper, card, fabric and can also be used as a glaze — see chapter 6)

You will notice that my list does not include Superglue; that is because I consider it to be very dangerous and overrated. It is only suitable for a limited range of uses, few of which have anything to do with making leisure equipment.

Other materials needed for specific projects are decribed in the instructions for making the piece of equipment.

It is easy to build up a collection of materials simply by keeping your eyes open when you are shopping and by thinking twice before you throw any packaging away. Plastic bottles, cardboard tubes and boxes, cellophane sweet wrappers, bubble plastic, the plasticized foil wrapping from some brands of biscuits and tea bags — all of these, and more, can be useful. The dedicated material-gatherer may even get to the stage of buying particular products because of their packaging!

Visit your local fabric shop or department regularly to see what interesting remnants they have; they should also be willing to sell you small lengths of fabric from the rolls (usually 20 cm is the minimum) and they may have scraps of ribbons, trimmings and odd buttons. Soft furnishing shops and departments will have remnants of heavier fabrics and trimmings. If you want a small piece of towelling, it is often cheaper to buy a small hand towel or face flannel than a length of fabric.

Make friends with your local charity shops. Clothes and cushion covers can often provide interesting textures, and they are fine once they are washed or dry cleaned. Some shops encourage dressmakers to donate leftover fabric and trimmings, which they then sell very cheaply.

Think about local shops and the companies and industries in your area — are they likely to be throwing out materials you could use? Printers often have spare paper and card, carpet warehouses have old samples, and the thick cardboard tubes from rolls of carpet, and so on. Searching for these materials is time-consuming. If you are lucky enough to have a scrapbank or play resource centre (see chapter 10) in your area, they will have done all the work for you and you should be able to become a member and have access to lots of lovely scrap materials.

Safety

There are two aspects of safety to consider: your safety when you are making the equipment, and the safety of anyone who is using it. Most, but not all, of the rules concerned with your safety apply to woodworking:

1. Before starting work
   — tie back long hair,
   — roll up loose sleeves,
   — remove jewellery, ties, scarves, anything which might get caught in a moving tool.
2. Treat all tools, hand or electric, with respect.
3. If you don't know how to use a tool, ask someone who does to show you how to use it and to stay with you until you are confident. Make sure you know how to turn power tools **off**.
4. Blunt tools are more dangerous than sharp ones. Replace the blades of a junior hacksaw or electric jigsaw regularly; use sharp craft knives. Tool shops should be able to sharpen twist drills for you.
5. Always wear safety spectacles or goggles when using tools.
6. Remember that drill bits and saw blades will be hot after use.
7. All electric tools must be used with a residual current circuit breaker; this will cut off the current if there is a fault in the tool or if the cable is damaged. The circuit breaker plugs into the wall socket and the tool plugs into the circuit breaker. If you have to use an extension lead (see below), plug the lead into the circuit breaker then the extension lead and anything plugged into it will be protected.
8. Work as close as possible to a socket, to avoid having trailing extension leads.
9. Always disconnect power tools when not in use and before changing drill bits, saw blades, or sheets of sandpaper.
10. Keep tools clean, brushing off sawdust after use. Ask a qualified electrician to check power tools regularly — cleaning the electrical contacts inside the tool, checking the cable and plug for signs of wear or damage, and so on.

11. Always work in good light, without distractions.
12. Use varnish, glues and spray mount in a well-ventilated area.

There are various points to consider when we look at the safety of the piece of equipment you have made:

1. Ensure that all surfaces and edges of wooden objects are smooth, and the corners rounded. Check that there are no splinters and no protruding nails or screws.
2. Ensure that all wood finishes are non-toxic:

    Varnish — polyurethane varnish (e.g. Ronseal) is safe and non-toxic once dry. Do not use yacht varnish (may contain chemicals) or coloured varnishes (stains used are toxic). **Paint** — use Humbrol enamel (available in small tins from model makers' shops) or gloss paints sold for use on toys; look for a statement 'meets the requirements of the European Safety Standard EN71 Part 3 1988 and BS5665 Part 3 1989' on the tin. Both enamel and gloss paint will need an undercoat. Apply two top coats, plus two coats of varnish for a really tough finish.

    You can also use ready mixed paints and poster paints (sold for use by children and therefore non-toxic). These won't need undercoat but they will need several coats of varnish to protect them. Yellow tends to be a bad pigment for covering the wood — try a coat of white under the yellow. These paints are useful for more detailed work such as painting features or patterns.

    A different effect can be produced by using drawing inks (make sure they are intended for use by children) or food colourings. These stain the wood, rather than coating it as paint does. These finishes will need several coats of varnish.
3. If the person is at the stage of exploring things with her mouth, make sure that removable parts are not small enough to be swallowed or wedged in the throat.
4. Do not use long-haired fur fabric if the item is likely to be mouthed, as the hairs are shed easily.
5. Any objects sewn onto a piece of equipment — ribbons, buttons, bells, etc. must be very firmly attached using strong thread. If you want to put eyes on the object, you can use safety eyes (available from craft shops) but it is probably safer to embroider the eyes or use scraps of felt. If you are attaching buttons, reinforce the back of the fabric with a piece of linen or calico, or place another button on the wrong side of the fabric so that you are sewing through button/fabric/button.

It is important to remember that there is no such thing as a completely safe piece of equipment — in the wrong hands, the most carefully designed and constructed object can be dangerous. Indeed, the sturdier you make the piece of equipment the more of a risk it will be if it is thrown or dropped on someone's foot.

There are some items which should be safe for unsupervised use and others which should be used by an enabler and the person with disabilities together, partly for safety reasons but also so that the person gets the maximum benefit and enjoyment from the activity.

Remember, also, that whilst we want most pieces of equipment to survive a reasonable length of time there is a place for the 'five minute item' — the puppet made out of a paper bag or a scrap of fabric, a simple jigsaw made from a picture mounted on card. These items are quickly made, often in the presence of the person who will use them, and can be enjoyed for as long as they last.

Another important point is that a safe piece of equipment will not necessarily remain safe for ever. Objects can get damaged in use — wood is knocked and chewed so that splinters and rough corners appear, screws work loose, seams start to come undone, and so on. It is essential to check equipment, both DIY and commercial, regularly and carry out any repairs so that the object survives and so, more importantly, does the user!

Many of the above comments apply equally to commercial equipment — the manufacturers set out to make items which are safe but they have no control over who uses them, and how. That is our responsibility.

Another aspect of safety which should not be overlooked is the use of batteries in leisure equipment. Batteries should always be inserted correctly, the battery compartment should be secured so that unauthorized people cannot get at the batteries, they should be removed when they are dead and disposed of in the bin (never in a fire or an incinerator).

If equipment is not going to be used for a while, remove batteries so that they won't leak or corrode the contacts. Always store batteries in a secure, dry place.

If you have popular battery powered items, it makes sense to use rechargeable batteries wherever possible. The initial outlay is very high but you will save a great deal of money in the long term, provided you train everyone not to throw the batteries away when they run down! Rechargeable batteries don't last as long between charges as the life you would get from ordinary batteries, so it is useful to have a spare set charged up, but of course that adds to the expense.

Always check the instructions to make sure you can use rechargeables — some pieces of equipment cannot stand the sudden surge of power from a freshly charged battery, nor the sudden stop when it runs out (ordinary batteries fade away). I find it helpful to stick a label on the lid of the battery compartment of such items to remind me not to use rechargeables.

Always charge batteries according to the instructions on your charger and in a safe place where they won't be disturbed. Never put ordinary batteries in a battery charger.

A few pieces of equipment use button cell batteries (the type used in watches and some hearing aids). These batteries are dangerous if swallowed — always make sure that the battery holder is sealed (with PVC tape if necessary) so that the batteries cannot fall out or be removed without your knowledge. Dispose of old batteries very carefully. When inserting new batteries, hold them with a paper tissue so that grease from your fingers doesn't get on the contacts.

Finding Other People to Make Equipment

It can be very enjoyable and satisfying to make equipment but you need facilities, skills and above all time to do it. For many of us it may make sense to find someone who is willing to make things. Organizing an equipment making project can be a highly successful, mutually beneficial exercise which produces useful and enjoyable leisure equipment or it can be a frustrating, time-consuming experience which results in unsuitable end products, or none at all. Here are a few guidelines which may help:

1. Be clear about what you want.
2. Check that the person has the necessary skills to make the item — difficult to assess, particularly if you don't have the skills yourself, but perhaps you could ask to see examples of their work?
3. Make sure that they are aware of all the safety requirements (paint, strong construction, size of pieces, etc.)
4. If the colour, texture, brightness of lights, loudness of sounds, etc. are important, say so.
5. Be clear about who will pay for materials — inability to provide them may deter individuals from offering to help and few schools and colleges can afford to make equipment unless the materials are paid for.
6. Agree a realistic date for delivery of the finished products — individual volunteers will have other commitments as well, but should be able to complete a project fairly quickly; schools and colleges may be looking for projects to last a term, or even an academic year, so it's no good asking them for something you want urgently!
7. Make sure you are asking the right person to carry out a particular project. If you need something designed to meet a need, you want someone who is interested in problem solving or a design student. If you have a worksheet, a set of instructions in a book, or a detailed description of the item required, you need someone who is willing (or is being trained) to follow instructions and not use their imagination.
8. And finally . . . be grateful! It is all too easy, in our busy lives, to receive the equipment, start using it and forget to write a 'thank you' letter.

So how do we find people to help us?

1. Women's, youth or church groups are often willing to save junk materials and make simple pieces of equipment.
2. Keen 'do-it-yourselfers' and unemployed or retired craftspeople may welcome the chance to use their skills — put posters up in libraries, doctors' surgeries, local shops and try to get an item in the local papers.
3. Workshops set up to train unemployed young people, or to offer sheltered employment often have a good range of machines and are keen to help local organizations and individuals.
4. Craft, design and technology teachers in schools are always looking for projects for their students.
5. Colleges need projects for their art and engineering students.

Remember the guidelines above, keep in contact with people while they are making things for you, encourage them to show you their work as it progresses (and possibly try out prototypes), show them you appreciate their efforts and you should end up with some useful, appropriate and enjoyable equipment.

And try to make time to produce a few things yourself — it's fun, satisfying and we all need creative play!

3

Mobiles and Other Hanging Things

Some mobiles are meant to be looked at and listened to, but not touched; others are intended to be handled, pulled, moved and bashed. It is important, for the safety of the user and of the mobile, to be clear which type of mobile you are dealing with!

Mobiles Out of Reach

Look for objects which will be attractive from a distance; think about the positioning of the mobile — if it consists of flat shapes hung vertically, then someone immediately beneath it will see very little of the shapes. A mobile which is intended to make sounds must be hung in a current of air or in a position where an enabler can reach it to set it in motion.

Craft shops sell many books full of ideas for making mobiles; here are a few simple ones to get you started:

1. Plastic cups, plain or painted, some with bells in and some with plastic beads (to form the 'clapper' of the bell).
2. Concave/convex mirrors and shapes cut from plastic mirrors (all available from the science section of education catalogues), to reflect the light.
3. Faulty compact discs (ask local stockists if they know of a source) make an ideal adult mobile, with plenty of movement and reflections.
4. 'Stained glass' mobiles — cut holes in pieces of stiff black paper (fold a square of paper in four, cut small shapes out of the folded edges to form a pattern when the paper is opened out). Stick coloured cellophane sweet wrappers over the holes and hang the mobile where the sun or a bright light will shine on it.
5. Make a mobile of balloons — ordinary rubber ones or metallic balloons. Stick on pieces of self-adhesive diffraction foil for added interest.
6. Fish mobile — cut circles out of gold and silver card, by drawing round a saucer or small plate. Cut into the middle of each circle, and overlap

the edges to make a slightly conical shape. Cut fins and trailing tails from diffraction foil wrapping paper (not self-adhesive). Staple round the edges of each pair of cones, to join them together, stapling fins and tails in position as appropriate. Cut out a 'V' shape to make a gaping mouth. These fish are very light and will move easily in the slightest breeze.

7. Convection snakes — cut circles of diffraction foil wrapping paper (not self-adhesive). Cut a spiral from each circle. Hang the spirals up by one end and they will move in the rising currents of warm air.

8. Cardboard tubes — paint spirals or apply coloured PVC tape in a spiral pattern. Hang the tubes so that they will rotate freely.

9. Paper plates — decorate them with paint, felt pens, coloured labels or scraps of self-adhesive diffraction foil. Hang some vertically and some horizontally, so that the mobile looks interesting from all directions.

10. Washing up liquid bottles — cut off the base, using a craft knife. Starting at the bottom, cut a spiral (using scissors) until you get to the 'shoulder' of the bottle. Paint the spirals with enamel paint or decorate with self-adhesive diffraction foil or glitter paper.

11. Make mobiles from natural materials — conkers, acorns, twigs, pine cones.

12. Make a 'drinks' mobile, using empty cans and coloured plastic bottles.

13. Use metal pan scourers to make a glittery mobile.

14. Open umbrellas, suspended upside down, can be a very effective decoration for a room. Use patterned, fabric-covered umbrellas or the Chinese paper ones.

15. Hang a black umbrella upside down and hang weather symbols from it — raindrops cut from diffraction foil, clouds, sun.

16. Buy ceramic mobiles from craft and gift shops. They make a beautiful sound but they are not strong enough to be handled.

Mobiles to Touch

If mobiles are meant to be handled, we must be careful that:

1. The objects are securely attached and are safe to be handled and mouthed.
2. The strings or cords are not so long that people can become entangled in them.
3. The mobile is securely fixed to an anchorage point which can stand the strain.

There are several commercial mobiles:

1. Hanging Chimeabout and Hanging Mirror Chimeabout (Edu-Play) — plenty of noise and movement when you pull the cord.
2. Bird mobiles (Mike Ayres & Co., Raven, Rompa, TFH, plus craft shops) — the wings flap gently when the cord is pulled.
3. Inflatable animals (joke shops) — large, brightly coloured and very light.

4. Brass windchimes (Mike Ayres & Co., Rompa) — beautiful sound, hang them where people can run their fingers through them.

You could also try:

1. Plastic Slinkies (toy shops) — usually have a fluorescent colour on one side and white on the other. Hang them up as unusual mobiles which will move easily when touched.
2. Parrot toys (pet shops) — a range of large bells and wooden shapes strung together on chains, which make an interesting mobile to handle.
3. Streamer Carousel — this design is from 'Make it Simple' by Carol Ouvry and Suzie Mitchell (The Consortium, 1990) and it is included here by kind permission of the authors. The mobile offers plenty of movement, bright colours and a wonderful rustling sound whenever it is disturbed. Carol and Suzie used hot air balloon material but I use kite fabric, as it is easier to obtain (from Brookite).

   Bind a plastic hoop with strips of a non-slippery material (this helps to stop the strips of kite fabric slipping round the hoop and making the mobile unbalanced). Tie a piece of string across the diameter of the hoop and a second piece across at right angles to the first. Knot another piece of string at the point where they cross, to suspend the mobile. Check that the cross is exactly in the middle of the circle and apply a spot of UHU or Bostik glue, to make sure it stays there.

   Cut strips of kite fabric 2 metres long. The width of the strips will depend on the size of your hoop — narrower for a small hoop, wider strips for a large one. The kite fabric has faint lines which make it easier to cut the strips. Fold each strip in half and attach to the hoop by wrapping the looped end round the hoop and pulling the two ends through the loop.

   The colours can be varied — all one colour, two contrasting colours, different sections, or mixed multicoloured strips. When the hoop is completely covered, hang it up and trim the ends. You can use different sized hoops, ranging from a small embroidery hoop to the largest size of plastic hoop, depending on the effect you want to achieve, and how much fabric you can afford!

Ways of Hanging Things

Individual objects described in the first section (above) can be hung up in various ways, to form a mobile:

1. Suspend the objects from a wire coathanger.
2. Tie two plant canes together to form a cross, and suspend objects from the ends and from the point where they cross.
3. Hang a plastic hoop horizontally and suspend objects all round it, making sure they are evenly balanced.
4. Make a classic balanced mobile, in which objects hang at different levels

and move in different directions, using lengths of thin cane. Make sure that each level is balanced and that the objects can move freely without hitting each other. Books on making mobiles will give you the layout for balanced mobiles.

5. Remove the fabric from an old umbrella, hang it upside down and hang objects from the framework.
6. Hang objects from a lampshade frame.
7. Buy a witch's hat (cheap ones are usually available at Halloween), hang it up by the point and suspend objects which will show up well against the black fabric.

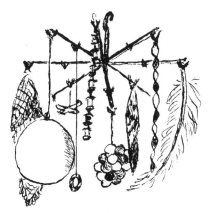

hung out of reach

8. Use a drip dry carousel (a plastic framework with spring pegs, sold in camping and hardware stores or from Lakeland Plastics) to hang various objects — feathers, balloons, sparkly jewellery, etc. for an out-of-reach mobile; chiffon scarves or scraps of fabrics for a mobile which can be touched.
9. Hang mobiles from a folding towel rail or from a retractable clothes line (the type which is usually fitted over a bath). These are not strong enough for mobiles which may be pulled, but they are useful because they can be stowed away when they are not needed.
10. Use 'Anywhere Hooks' (suction hooks which will stick to any smooth, non-porous surface; usually displayed with travel goods) to hang objects against a wall or window, or tie a length of thin cord between two hooks to support light mobiles.
11. Use a travel clothes line (from camping shops), which consists of a double elastic twisted and with a hook at each end. Push objects between the elastic, wherever you want them to hang.
12. Fix a length of curtain wire across the room, at ceiling height or along a beam, by stretching the wire between two hooks secured in the walls. If it is a long length, support the wire in the middle with another hook.

Never hang mobiles, however lightweight, from light fittings.

The problem with many mobiles is that the strings easily become tangled when the objects move in the breeze. Leon Charman, a classroom assistant at the RNIB Sunshine House School in Northwood, has a simple solution. When you are making the mobile, thread each string through a length of thin, transparent plastic tubing. The plastic hardly shows but it will stop the strings tangling.

Remember that mobiles don't have to hang from the ceiling: choose an attractive branch, wedge it in a pot or tub using stones and fill with Polyfilla to hold it firmly in place. Hang pine cones, dried flowerheads, feathers, green lamella foil. At Christmas, decorate the branch with battery powered tree lights and hang baubles and silver foil.

Objects which are meant to be touched and pulled must be very securely anchored:

1. Use a sturdy hook screwed into a joist in the ceiling.
2. Screw a length of slotted metal from a shelving system (Spur or similar) onto the wall. Use the largest bracket available (so that the mobile will hang clear of the wall) and attach the mobile to it.
3. Tie strong plastic netting (from garden centres) at a suitable height for someone to lie underneath it. Hang various objects from the netting. When the person knocks or pulls one of the objects, the rest will bounce up and down.
4. Hang a mobile from an indoor netball goalpost, with the base weighted with sand or water.
5. A garden parasol (with the base weighted with sand or water) may be used indoors or outside. You can leave the fabric on the parasol (provided the objects will show up clearly against the pattern). If you remove the fabric, glue a wooden bead or a small rubber ball on the end of each spoke to avoid eye injuries.
6. A rotary clothes line can be used to suspend mobiles when people are outside — hang objects to be pulled on the metal arms and bells, tinsel, etc. out of reach on the clothes line.

Whatever type of mobiles you make or buy, remember to change them around frequently and introduce new ones — a mobile which has been hanging in the same place for a few months will be about as exciting as the wallpaper!

4

Sensory Stimulation

Sight

Vision is our main co-ordinating sense, helping us to understand our world and the things that are happening around us. In recent years there has been a great deal of research into the development of vision in new-born babies and infants and we now know a lot about the way babies see, and what attracts them visually.

It is impossible to know exactly what a person with profound disabilities can see, but if there is a very severe developmental delay it seems logical to assume that the development of vision has also been affected. An understanding of how vision develops may therefore help us to offer visual stimulation which is relevant, interesting and non-threatening.

At birth, a baby can only see clearly objects which are about 20 cm from her eyes; this increases to about 30 cm by the time she is six weeks old. During her first two months she can see differences in shape, size and pattern. She will prefer high contrast patterns (black and white) to colours, and fairly complex patterns. When the baby looks at her mobile she will be more interested in the outside edge of each shape than the pattern on it.

By about two months the baby can scan the entire visual field. She will explore both the shape of an object and its surface decoration. She will prefer curved shapes to angular ones and be attracted to faces and complex patterns such as bullseye or chessboard patterns.

At about four months the baby can adjust her focus to see both near and distant objects and she can see in full colour.

When we are working on visual stimulation, we should remember that visual awareness develops in the following sequence:

brightness and darkness, contrast
movement
shape
colour

Our visual effects are more likely to attract attention, for instance, if they incorporate movement. Bold contrast is much more important than pretty colours.

Here is a collection of ideas for visual stimulation; some of them will be successful in daylight, others need a dark room. Where reference is made to a spotlight, you could use a bright torch or an anglepoise light instead.

Lights

1. Lullaby Light Show (Tomy) — the dome rotates, as the music plays, and projects coloured shapes onto the ceiling. If you feel that the animal shapes are childish, partly cover them with small pieces of self-adhesive labels so that abstract shapes are lit up. If the person cannot look at the ceiling, or the room is not dark enough, there are other ways you can use the Light Show.

   Line a large cardboard box with foil and stand it on its side, facing the person. Place the Light Show in the box, so that the lights shine on the foil. Alternatively, cut a circle in the 'roof' of the box and place the Light Show on top of the box, upside down, with the dome fitting through the hole.

   Drape the person with a white sheet, place the Light Show in her lap and position her in front of a large mirror.

2. Fibre optic torches — cheap torches (about £2) are sometimes available in shops and on market stalls. When switched on, coloured lights appear at the end of the fibre optic strands. They are particularly effective in a dark room and can be stroked gently on the skin or waved back and forth. The strands are quite hard and easily broken and you may be concerned that they will be poked in someone's eye or put in the mouth. If you want to be able to let people handle the torch without anxiety, choose the fibre optic torch supplied by Kirton Litework. It is more expensive (about £10), but the strands are so soft that they cannot be broken and they would cause no more harm in the eye than an eyelash.

3. Have a selection of torches, particularly ones with interchangeable coloured lenses. These are available quite cheaply, and have two, three or four colours. Look for torches with faces on the lens. The Thomas the Tank Engine Torch looks childish, but it projects a clear, simple face on the wall.

4. Motorists' lamps (the cylindrical type) have red and orange bulbs (sometimes flashing) and a fluorescent light which you can put your hands round. Some lamps can be used with a battery adaptor and pressure switch (see chapter 7), so that people can switch them on unaided.

5. Disco Visor or Headband with flashing lights (some shops, or TFH) — either you wear it and the person looks at you, or she wears it and looks in a mirror. You could also use a flashing bow tie (from joke and novelty shops).

6. Some cycle shops sell right and left indicators for cyclists — an orange light which straps to the wrist and flashes when the arm is raised.

7. Place sweet wrappers, scraps of tissue paper and pieces of acetate on the

sticky side of self-adhesive clear plastic and stick it on the window for the sun to shine through.

8. Hang stained-glass roundels and crystals (from gift catalogues and shops) or faceted Christmas baubles in the window to catch the sunlight.

9. Use a transparent water tray in a dark room. Colour the water with food colouring, shine a spotlight on it and let the water run through a colander or cutlery drainer.

10. Shine a spotlight through Leybourne Colour Frames (from Mike Ayres & Co.)

11. Shine a spotlight on a clear PVC ball (Mike Ayres & Co., Rompa) containing coloured balls. Add water for sloshing noises and pieces of silver foil for more visual effect.

12. Battery-powered Christmas-tree lights — safe, because they operate on very low voltage and the 'bulbs' are LEDs, not glass bulbs. Some sets only flash, others can be on continuously or flashing. They can be used in many ways, but the wires are vulnerable to damage and tangling, so you might like to make them into a light board.

Light Board

This idea was given to me by Martha Tomkin, who is a home manager at Ravenswood Village. I haven't seen the one Martha made, so I don't know how she did it, but this is my version.

The light board uses hardboard the 'wrong way round'. The front of the board is the rough side (usually the underside) of the hardboard, because it is a good matt surface for the lights. The smooth side, which is hidden inside the finished object, is a suitable surface for the PVC tape to stick to.

You will need two pieces of hardboard, about 30 cm × 35 cm, and a set of thirty battery-powered Christmas-tree lights (if you have a bigger set, you may wish to make a bigger board).

Mark where you want the lights to be on the rough side of one of the pieces of hardboard, leaving a border of 3 cm all round the board. The lights can be arranged in a pattern, or randomly. Place the hardboard, rough side uppermost, on a piece of scrap wood and drill the holes for the lights. The scrap wood will help to stop the hardboard breaking away as you drill the holes. Choose a drill which will allow the LED to pass through, but not the base of the light — I used a 6.2 mm drill, but you will have to find the correct size for your lights. Smooth the surface round each hole, using a file or sandpaper.

Pin (using panel pins) and glue lengths of 18 mm square section wood to three sides of the board, on the smooth side. Cut the wood for the fourth side slightly shorter, so that there is a small gap for the wires to pass through. Position the second piece of hardboard, smooth side out, on the top of the wood. Mark the position for the screws in each corner. Remove the hardboard and drill the holes, using a 3.0 mm drill. Countersink the holes slightly. Replace the hardboard and drill four

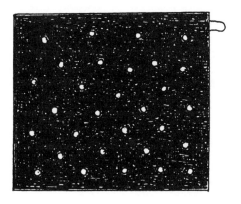

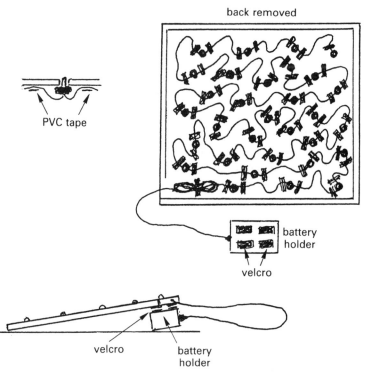

small holes (using a 1.5 mm drill) in the wood, below the holes in the hardboard. Don't go very far with these holes, they are only there to help the screws go into the wood. Screw down the hardboard, using 1/2 inch No. 6 countersunk screws. Remove the screws and put them and the hardboard safely to one side.

Paint the rough side of the top piece of hardboard and the outside edges of the wood with dark grey primer, then matt black paint (used for blackboards, available from DIY stores). When the paint is dry, rest the board (face down) on four cotton reels or small blocks of wood, so that you can poke the LEDs through and work on the back of the board.

Poke the first LED through the hole furthest away from the corner where you left the gap for the wires. Tape the wire down on either side of the light, using PVC insulation tape. Continue in this way until all the lights are in place. Use more PVC tape to anchor down any loose wires, if necessary. Anchor the last part of the wire securely with PVC tape, just inside the gap in the wood and leaving enough wire free for the battery compartment to be positioned in the middle of one of the long sides of the board. Screw the hardboard back in position.

Stick two or four (depending on the size of the battery holder) pieces of self-adhesive Velcro to the battery holder and the corresponding pieces of Velcro to the hardboard, in the middle of one of the long sides. Attach the battery holder and switch on.

The board can be held, propped up (on the battery holder) or laid flat (remove the battery holder and lie it beside the board).

13. Overhead projector — this can be used in so many ways for light stimulation. It can be positioned close to a wall, for a small bright light, or further away. A trolley will make it easier to position the OHP where you want it, or a piece of wood on castors, if you want ground level effects. Shine the light on the floor, ceiling or a hanging piece of net curtain. Move the beam from side to side and up and down. Use the inner sleeve from an LP record to make a smaller circle of light.

Various coloured effects can be produced using coloured OHP acetates, acetate from disco and theatre suppliers or coloured sweet wrappers. Make patterns of Octons (from Galt) which are transparent and beautiful colours.

The balls from various washing liquids (Ariel, Persil, etc.) come in different colours — orange, red, blue. Roll them on the OHP (or put them over the lens of a torch). Other transparent coloured objects can be rolled and spun on the OHP — try 'cut glass' plastic dishes, acrylic threading beads, car headlamps and indicator glass or coloured lens covers for pool lights. Cover the surface of the OHP with a sheet of clear acetate, taped down, to protect it when spinning or rolling objects.

14. Slide projectors — a good source of bright light for making shadows or spotlighting objects. Place a mirror in the beam and move it to shine the light around the room (not in people's eyes). Blow bubbles across the beam of light. Buy plastic slide casings and make your own set of colour slides, using different colours of acetate.

Draw a basic face shape on one; on others make black shapes by sticking small circular self-adhesive labels and irregular shapes on the acetate (you can do this on a larger scale with the OHP, using sheets of coloured acetate). Create white shapes by making small holes in the acetate. Shine these coloured patterns on the wall, people and objects.

15. Visual stimulation videos — there are several computer programmes which offer exciting visual images, but not everyone has access to a computer. What is needed is a range of videos which offer similar visual stimulation, since many more people have a television and video machine. Some videos have been produced, using computer graphics transferred to video, and linking the images to music (see chapter 11). More videos are needed.

Reflections and Glitter

1. Place a crumpled survival blanket on top of a mat or mattress. The person lying on this will hear the rustling and see the reflections as she moves. This should be used under supervision, as there is a very slight risk of suffocation.

2. Hologram badges and brooches with flashing lights (gift shops and catalogues) are fun to look at and wear.

3. Laser discs (gift shops and catalogues) are metal discs covered with diffraction foil. A 'dimple' on the underside ensures that the disc spins easily and the reflections are beautiful (especially under a spotlight). You can produce the same effect on a larger scale by sticking a circle of diffraction foil to a 'Lazy Susan'. You can also stick various three-dimensional shapes covered in foil and glitter papers round the edge of the 'Lazy Susan', which will reflect the light as it spins.

4. Make a mobile using bicycle reflectors and safety stickers (sold for children's coats) and shine a spotlight on it.

5. Shine lights on Indian cushion covers which incorporate mirrors in the embroidery.

6. Glitter pompoms (from Toys'R'Us, for American football cheerleaders) produce a wonderful glitter effect when waved in a bright light. Gold and silver are best but they are getting more difficult to obtain, the coloured ones are attractive but not so effective. You could make your own with a survival blanket, a sharp pair of scissors — and a lot of patience !

7. Stick pieces of self-adhesive Velcro 'loops' to the inside surface of a projection tent (Kirton Litework). Hang various shiny objects — inflated wine bag, unbreakable Christmas tree baubles, parrot bells, sequinned motifs (flowers, butterflies — from haberdashery shops and craft fairs), tinsel, etc. Place mats and cushions in the tent, so that the person can lie in comfort and look at the decorations.

8. Buy ruffled hair decorations — some already have gold, silver and 'jewels' on them, others can have bells securely attached. Wear them round ankles or wrists.

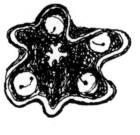 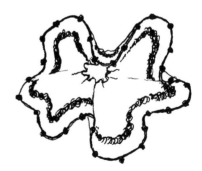

9. Collect the clear plastic tubes with stoppers which contain small chocolates or sugared almonds. Place assorted sequins in one, small 'glass' beads (sold for embroidery) in another and coloured foil lamella in

a third. These tubes aren't for tough guys, but they are light and easy to wave around. The lamella provides a particularly useful filling because it makes no sound, so if the person looks at it she is doing so because she can see it, not because she is turning towards a sound.

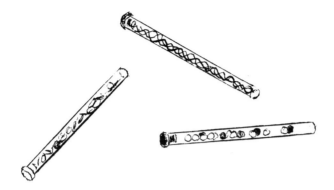

10. The Pat Mat (SNC Playring) consists of a plastic pillow with two handles. The base is opaque white and the top is clear plastic. It contains foam shapes of fish, crabs, starfish and other creatures. When the Pat Mat is filled with water the shapes move around as the mat is patted. It is best to use distilled water (it will stay clean longer) and always use both handles when you are lifting the mat — water is very heavy and will place a strain on the welding at one end of the mat, if you don't.

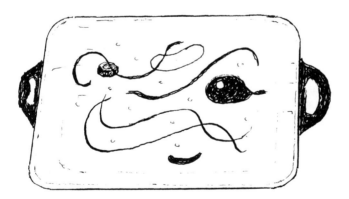

The coloured foam shapes are attractive, but much more visual stimulation can be achieved if you remove them (through the plug for the water) and insert fluorescent shoelaces, shapes cut from diffraction foil wrapping paper (not self-adhesive) and survival blanket, and shapes cut from thin black PVC. You could also add glitter (but you will probably never get it all out again) or food colouring (but this may stain the white plastic base after a while). Use the mat under a spotlight, for best effect.

11. Tocki tubes (see chapter 11) are wonderful glitter tubes made of clear acrylic plastic and filled with a non-toxic mineral oil. They contain glitter, coloured granules and sequins which cascade down the tube. The tubes can be enjoyed individually but there is also a sturdy hardwood frame which holds four tubes and a kaleidoscope which creates visually stimulating effects from the movement of the tube's contents.

12. Attach foil streamers to the wire casing of a fan, or blow the fan through a foil streamer curtain — make your own from a survival blanket, or buy one from a novelty shop (e.g. Barnum's).

13. Fill a bowl full of silver lamella, or cut up survival blanket — for rummaging.

14. Use shiny baking tins, stainless steel dog bowls and metal colanders for 'putting in and taking out' games.

Contrast

1. Stim-Mobile (SNC Playring) — a plastic mobile with vertical and horizontal surfaces decorated with simple and complex patterns in black and white. Also available: Pattern Play — soft vinyl 'cards' which can be held, hung up or linked together to form a book; and Double Feature — a large (41 cm × 30.5 cm) acrylic mirror with bold black and white images on the reverse.

2. Make your own black and white materials:
   - pompoms of black streamers (rubbish sacks) and white (swing bin bags)
   - black and white chiffon scarves, or net curtain (plain and dyed black)
   - paper plates decorated with black felt pens, black PVC tape or shapes cut out of black Fablon
   - black and white balloons
   - plastic beads and bangles
   - strips of black and white plastic tied to the wire cage of a fan.

3. Make a visual stimulation mat:

   Make a mat using black velvet and polyester wadding (see the Noughts and Crosses Board in chapter 8 for the method). Attach various objects which will give a good contrast against the black:
   - Child's sock, in fluorescent green — place a flat squeaker (from craft shops) in the toe of the sock. Pin across the line from the point where the heel turns. Place a strip of bubble plastic, folded in four, in the leg of the sock and oversew the opening. Machine the sock to the mat along the line of pins.
   - Pearl buttons with irridescent flecks — arrange in a pattern and sew on firmly, using strong button thread.
   - Bottle — choose a clean, dry cylindrical bottle and place some dry rice inside. Cut a strip of white towelling to fit round the bottle. Machine black ric-rac braid in diagonal stripes across the towelling.

Place a length of piping cord down the side of the bottle, underneath, and up the other side of the bottle, securing it with PVC tape. Sew the towelling round the bottle. Cut two circles of towelling, slightly larger than the ends of the bottle. Turn under the raw edges and sew them on, making sure that the ends of the piping cord are sticking out and that you stitch through the cord as you sew on the top circle. Sew the piping cord to the mat.

- Net flower — concertina fold a strip of fluorescent net. Hold firmly in the middle and gently pull the folds round to form a rosette. Pin through all the thicknesses to the mat. Sew white buttons in the centre of the rosette, arranging them in a pattern and using them to catch down all the layers of the net. Remember to remove all the pins — it is easy to miss them in the net.
- Clacker — buy a child's fluorescent clacker toy. Cut off the handle (below the first flange, so that the clackers stay on the rod), using a junior hacksaw. Sew firmly to the mat, using black carpet thread, at either end of the rod. Make sure that the clackers can still swing freely.
- Streamers — cut strips of fluorescent kite fabric (from Brookite). Tie them in a knot in the centre. Arrange on the mat and machine across all the streamers on either side of the knot.
- Machine loops of black tape to the mat and tie on a small white sieve, alternate large black and white buttons on a strong piece of elastic, and two white rubber doorstops.

Fluorescence

Fluorescent colours are five to eight times brighter than ordinary colours. Under ultraviolet (UV) light, they become thirty times more visible. However, there are some concerns about the use of UV light, and no clear guidelines. The UV light must be diffuse and the source shielded, and sessions should be limited to 15 minutes. However, an enabler working in short sessions with several people will have been exposed for much longer than the recommended time. Many of the fluorescent effects suggested below are very effective under a bright spotlight and it may be sensible to do this rather than use UV.

1. Fluorescent paints, inks, felt pens and modelling materials can be used for art and craft activities.
2. Fluorescent tape and self-adhesive paper labels can be used to highlight objects and surfaces.
3. Make streamers from strips of fluorescent kite fabric.
4. Use fluorescent sun block (from ski shops) to highlight parts of the face, fingers, etc.
5. Put fluorescent paint in a strong plastic bag, tape the end closed with PVC tape and tape it flat on the table — an interesting squidgy texture.

6. Dress up in fluorescent fashion wear and bicycle safety gear.
7. Balsac Balloon Ball (toy shops, Rompa) — a large balloon which is blown up inside a thin cotton bag. All the bags are patterned, some are fluorescent. You could also make plain covers, or attach textures to the bag. If you place coins between the bag and the balloon as you inflate it, the ball will roll in an interesting way. Dry rice or lentils inside the balloon will produce a noise. The balloon ball is particularly useful for situations in which the use of balloons has been banned (because of the danger of swallowing pieces of rubber if the balloon bursts). The bag protects the balloon from bursting, but if it does burst, the pieces of rubber are safely inside the bag.

Sound

We use our sense of hearing before we are born; in the womb the baby can hear the sounds of her mother's body and voice and noises from the world outside. By the time they are born, most babies prefer female voices and, within a few weeks, the baby can recognize the sound of her mother's speech.

Many people with profound disabilities have some degree of hearing impairment, they often have problems making sense of verbal communication and difficulty making sounds of their own. Helping people to develop an awareness of sound may enable them to make sense of their surroundings, lead to the enjoyment of particular sounds and the ability to indicate preferences.

Music should play an important part in any 'sounds' work we do, and various suppliers of musical instruments are listed in chapter 11. It is also possible to make musical instruments, but we must be careful — too often people with disabilities are given home-made shakers, drums, etc., and denied access to real musical instruments. Shortage of funds is no justification for giving people equipment we would not want to use ourselves. Rather than spending ages hunting for materials and making 'instruments' which produce unsatisfactory or unpleasant noises, our time would be better spent persuading budget holders of the need for equipment, or for more imaginative spending of clients' money, or organizing a leisure library so that available equipment can be shared, or fund-raising for musical instruments.

Here are some ideas for using sounds and music:

1. Look in toy shops, craft shops and catalogues for wooden bell cubes and rattles which are not childish.
2. Last Christmas, I found a large (about 10 cm diameter) red sleigh bell which makes a lovely sound and you can feel the vibration of the ball moving around inside.
3. Craft books always recommend buying budgerigar bells, but I find they don't make much noise. However, pet shops sell parrot bells, which are

big and noisy. Edu-Play sell smaller bells which make a satisfactory sound.

4. Bell Carousel/Round Bells (Early Learning Centre, Raven) — a circle of bells with clear, pure notes. It spins easily and a beater held in the way will produce a peal of bells. TFH sell a motorized version, which can be operated by a switch, for people who cannot spin or hit the bells.

5. Sounds Mat — TFH sell one, ACTIVE (see chapter 10) publish a worksheet to make one. Any movement on the mat, or pressing the pads, produces various sounds.

6. A battery-operated whisk, or a fan or hairdryer, will produce sound and air.

7. Collect musical birthday and Christmas cards, which play tunes when they are opened (some have little LED lights as well).

8. Look for musical mugs which play a tune when lifted and stop when they are put down.

9. Sound story books (toy and book shops) — some of the stories, especially the Disney ones, are acceptable. Pressing various pads produces sounds which link in with the story.

10. Sound books (bookshops) — pressing a button produces the sound of a siren, bird, frog, etc. (depending on the story). The stories are not suitable but you can stick new pages over the original ones, with appropriate words and pictures or photographs.

11. Tape recordings of natural sounds (sea, rain, birds, etc.) are available — see chapter 11.

12. Make your own tape recordings of special events or outings and make a book of photographs, entrance tickets, leaflets, etc. to look at.

13. Record sound stories, using everyday sounds. Sound effects tapes and records are available, for a wider range of source material.

14. Place beads or pasta shapes on an upturned tambour; they will roll around and jump when the tambour is hit from below.

15. Make sounds together — clapping hands, tapping objects (with finger, hand or another object). Experiment with different rhythms and objects — hollow, solid, large, small, plastic, wood.

16. Use the sounds the person makes — copy them, extend and combine them, use them as communication in a conversation, add movements.

17. Use a tape recorder to record people's sounds. Some people may find this threatening, but they are more likely to enjoy it and gain confidence because their sounds are being valued.

18. Make sounds by crumpling tissue paper, newspaper, glossy magazines, survival blanket.

19. Tear paper rhythmically to music — make a lovely mess, collect it up and have an outing to a recycling point.

20. Make up 'songs without words', using consonant or vowel sounds.

21. Rock together to the rhythm of the music — either side by side or facing each other and holding hands.

22. If you think the person has a hearing impairment, look for sounds which vibrate. A guitar or tongue drum (a wooden drum, from Acorn

Percussion or Knock on Wood) vibrate when they are played. Let the person lean against you, so that she can feel the vibration in your chest when you speak or sing. Rest your jaw against the bony ridge behind her ear as you talk, hum or sing.

23. Philips Sound Switch — this is a sound sensitive switch which will switch on a light when it detects a noise (sold as a burglar deterrent). Both the sound sensitivity and the length of time the light comes on for can be adjusted. Much cheaper (about £15) than interactive equipment sold by the specialist suppliers. Use it to encourage hand clapping, dropping objects or vocal sounds.

24. Use music selectively, not as a permanent background. If you talk to someone who has a degree of hearing loss, they will tell you how annoying background music is in shops, pubs and restaurants, because it stops them hearing the important things.

25. Match the music to the mood — Waterloo station plays lively music in the mornings and quiet relaxing music in the evenings when people are going home after a hard day's work.

26. Don't impose your taste in music — offer a wide range of musical styles. There are some suggestions in chapter 11.

27. Offer a wide range of musical instruments from different countries — suppliers of multicultural instruments are listed in chapter 11.

28. Soundbeam (see chapter 11) — this is an exciting piece of equipment which enables people with very little movement to play music. Any movement within the invisible ultrasonic beam 'plays' the electronic keyboard. New developments enable Soundbeam to be linked to various multisensory effects or to a vibrating board.

29. Personal stereo — this is a useful piece of equipment because it allows the individual to listen to music without interrupting other people or being interrupted. However, they are very vulnerable to damage and they dislike being dropped, thrown or trodden on. Martha Tomkin, from Ravenswood Village, solved this problem in the following way: take a 'bumbag' (a pouch for wearing round the waist when walking or cycling), cut a piece of foam plastic to fit in the bag. Using a sharp knife and care, cut a slot in the foam into which the stereo will fit, on its side with the controls uppermost. Close the zip carefully, with the leads coming out of the bag at the end of the zip.

Here are some DIY ideas for things to make:

Slither Box (Roma Lear)

This design appears in 'Play Helps'. You will need a sturdy, flat box (like a fancy chocolate box). Place a cupful of aquarium gravel inside and cover the box with Fablon (woodgrain effect looks good) for speed, or layers of papier mâché if you've got more time and want to make the box stronger. Use it for a seaside theme (waves on the shore) or for sound stories (walking on a gravel path). One of the best things about the slither box is the feeling of weight being transferred from one end of the box to the other as you tip it.

The next two items use Touch'n'Play Music Buttons, which are sold by The Craft Depot (see chapter 11). A good range of tunes is available (not just children's songs and lullabies) — 'Love Story', 'Send in the Clowns' and 'Somewhere my Love' for example. Christmas tunes are also available.

Musical Mat (JD)

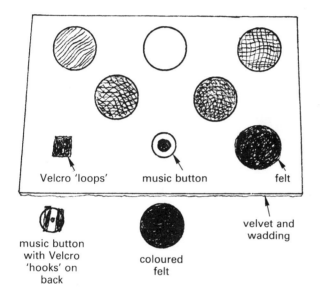

Velcro 'loops'   music button   felt

music button
with Velcro
'hooks' on
back

coloured
felt

velvet and
wadding

Make a mat approximately 25 cm x 30 cm using plain, dark fabric (e.g. black velvet) and a single layer of polyester wadding (see instructions for Noughts and Crosses mat in chapter 8). Don't make the mat too thick and soft because you need a firm surface to press the music buttons against. Sew eight pieces of Velcro 'loops' to the mat, either randomly or in a pattern.

Stick two small pieces of self-adhesive Velcro 'hooks' on the back of each button, on either side of the hole (if you stick Velcro over this hole you will muffle the sound). Cut circles of felt, 8 cm in diameter, in eight different colours. Place the buttons on the Velcro and sew a felt circle over each button, either by hand or using zig-zag stitch on the machine. Save the squares of felt (see below). Felt is ideal for this project because there is no problem of raw edges and good bright colours are available. Felt isn't washable, but then neither are the music buttons!

When the music mat needs cleaning, remove the felt and the buttons, wash or dry clean the mat (depending on the fabric you used), replace the buttons and cut new circles of felt from the squares you saved. Sew the circles on, ideally keeping the same colour as before for each tune so that people can find their favourites.

If dribbling is a problem, you could use PVC fabric for the circles or cover each button with clingfilm before adding the Velcro. But remember that the more layers, or the thicker they are, the more muffled the sound will be.

Musical Presents

Make a Christmas stocking out of red felt. Make various small 'presents' using scraps of fabric and trimmings. Place a music button (Christmas tunes) in each present and stuff lightly with polyester stuffing, working it into the corners and round the button.

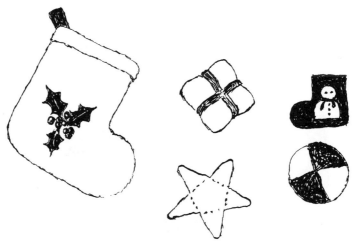

You could make a small wallhanging of a Christmas tree in green felt or baize, sew Velcro 'hook' pieces on the tree and 'loop' pieces on the presents. The presents can then be taken out of the stocking and put on the tree — you are almost certain to press the button in the process!

Touch

Touch is not just about textures — it also includes things which are hot or cold, vibration and the movement of air. All of these sensations are detected by our skin; we decide whether they are pleasant or not, and react accordingly.

Texture

This section starts with some simple ideas and then gives fuller descriptions of some pieces of equipment which can be made.

1. Rub body lotion on hands, arms, legs, etc. naming the body part as you do so.

2. Place sand, rice pudding, lentils or thick paint inside rubber gloves and tie the ends securely.

3. Fill pillowcases with autumn leaves, crumpled paper, foam offcuts, polystyrene packing shapes, crumpled survival blanket, tennis balls.

4. Make a collection of chains. DIY stores usually have a good selection — bath-plug chain, white plastic (for gardens), decorative gilt (for hanging lights etc.) and metal chains with different sizes and shapes of links. Fix them firmly to a board, for fiddling with, or provide a metal bowl for 'in and out' activities. Make your own chain, using large wooden rings (stained ones for curtain poles or plain ones from pet shops) and hinged rings (sold in stationers — put a dab of Araldite on the opening and the hinge). You could also use the nylon clips sold in yachting shops.

5. Buy a pair of brightly-coloured or fluorescent tights. Stuff the legs with cellophane, bubble plastic and Mylar (from metallic balloons). Tie a knot in the body of the tights. Place the tights round the neck, with the legs dangling down the front, so that the person has something to explore with her hands, plus the noise when she moves her head.

6. 'Tactile Stories: A Do-It-Yourself Guide to Making 6 Tactile Books'. This book, by Chris Fuller (published by The Consortium), provides instructions for making the props needed to tell a simple story, and the large, laminated story cards. The end product is the separate pages of the story, which can be taken round the group, rather than a conventional book. The stories incorporate smell and sound, as well as texture. They are simple, but not particularly childish and the ideas can be easily adapted to make your own stories.

7. There are very few good tactile books on the market (mainly because they are expensive to produce) and they are, understandably, aimed at children. There used to be some good books (with acceptable stories) which incorporated patterns of raised dots, but these are now out of print. Of course, you can make your own using fabrics, self-adhesive Vivelle (from Rompa) and the various products sold by RNIB for making raised markings. The pages of the book can be thick card, thin plywood or fabric.

8. Make 'necklaces' for people to wear and explore. Thread plastic shapes, wooden beads and rings, plastic pan scrubbers, etc. onto a length of thick piping cord or dressing gown cord.

9. Remember that it is important to feel harsh textures as well as soft ones (indeed, many people actually prefer them). You could make a large tactile wall board with mop heads, the pads from rotary floor scrubbers, brush heads, rubber mats, pieces of carpet, loofahs, green plastic 'grass' doormats and bristle doormats.

10. Some people won't explore if you give them a texture cushion or mat to touch, so turn the idea inside out! Make a bag of plain fabric and attach textures, bells, buttons, etc. to the *inside*. The person can sit with her hands in the bag and she will be feeling the textures however little she moves her hands. Alternatively you can leave both ends of the bag open to form a tube, like an old-fashioned muff. You could try the same idea with a foot muff. Sew textures all over the inside, but only attach bells to

the top surface — it could be very uncomfortable to have a bell under your foot.

Texture Mat (Sarah Lloyd)

Sarah made this mat when she was studying on the RNIB's in-service training course at Condover Hall School, which caters for multiply-disabled and deaf-blind students.

Choose four textured fabrics — velvet, corduroy, fur fabric and towelling, for example. Machine squares (approximately 50 cm) together to form a mat. Machine Velcro 'loops' to the centre of each square — use three 9 cm pieces of 3 cm wide Velcro, side by side, to make a large square. Make a large shape out of each fabric — cube, cylinder, heart and triangle, for example — by cutting out the required shapes, machining Velcro 'hooks' to the right side of one piece of fabric and machining the pieces together, leaving a gap in the final seam. Turn right side out and stuff each shape with polyester stuffing, foam chips or cut-up tights; slipstitch the seam closed.

People can lie on the mat to feel the textures, or use it on a table. Each shape can be matched to the appropriate square and attached to the Velcro.

Sensory Mat (Chia Swee Hong)

Chia Swee Hong is an occupational therapist in Norwich, and he suggests this variation on a texture mat.

Make a mat from four large pieces of textured materials — fur fabric, velvet, silky and lurex, for instance. Make it large enough for people to lie on. Make the following shapes:

cylinder	make a cylinder from each of the fabrics, 30 cm long and 10 cm in diameter; stuff with polyester stuffing.
square	cut four shapes, 30 × 10 × 10 cm, from foam plastic, using a serrated bread knife.
triangle	cut two shapes, 30 × 10 × 10 cm, from foam plastic. Cut them in half, lengthwise on the diagonal of the square, so that you have four pieces 30 cm long with a triangular cross-section.
rectangle	cut four shapes, 30 × 10 × 15 cm, from foam plastic.

Make covers for the squares, triangles and rectangles, using the four fabrics, so that you have one square covered in each of the textures, and so on.

The finished item can be used in various ways:

1. Lie on the mat and feel the textures.
2. Match the blocks according to texture.
3. Match the blocks according to shape.

4. Match the blocks to the textures on the mat.
5. Build a tower of blocks and knock them down.

Tactile Carpet (Caroline Allen)

This mat was designed by Caroline, who is Deputy Head at Orchard Hill
Further Education Centre.

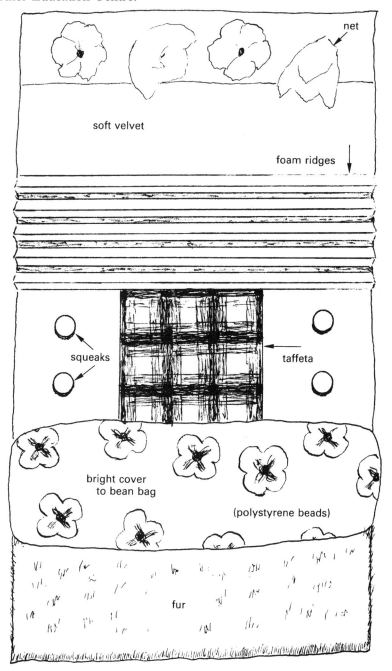

She writes:

During sessions which focus on sensory stimulation I have often used small objects for tactile experiences. However, I thought that the students might benefit from a large scale tactile object which could be in contact with several parts of the body at once. I thought of the idea of a 'tactile carpet' as a large size tactile experience like the vibrating bed or jacuzzi, but as a potentially more versatile piece of equipment offering a variety of tactile stimuli.

Many large pieces of equipment have limited use because they are difficult to move around. I decided to design the carpet so that it could roll up and be used in any room.

The carpet is designed to tempt the student to move on to the next section. I did not design it with any one student in mind, although I initially conceived of it in terms of the students on the sensory discrimination taster course. I realised that students from other groups could benefit; for example, Freddie might crawl along it from end to end, Susan might discover it stretched across tables encouraging her to reach forward and explore, Stephen might feel it on the wall like a wallhanging, enticing him to reach up and stand upright.

Landscape Mat (JD)

This mat was, believe it or not, inspired by driving along the M40 motorway! In late spring and early summer the patchwork of fields presents an incredible range of colours — the brown of ploughed earth, green grass and crops, yellow flowers of oil-seed rape, beige hay — and I wondered if it would be possible to make a tactile mat which looked like an aerial photograph of the countryside.

Take a piece of calico, about 150 cm x 100 cm and tack a line all round, 2 cm from the edge. Cut an irregular shape from a brown fabric, to form a hill in the centre of the mat. Machine the fabric to the mat, leaving some fullness and a small gap in the seam. Stuff the hill with polyester stuffing — not too firmly, or it will pull the base fabric up too much.

Now work out a patchwork arrangement of fields, working outwards from the slopes of the hill. Make the fields square, rectangular and other angular shapes and introduce as many different textures as possible. All the colours should be shades of green, brown and yellow so that they look as realistic as possible. My fields are made of fabric and knitting:

velvet
towelling
velour
needlecord
elephant cord (very thick corduroy)
quilted fabric
fur fabric

green foam carpet underlay
green pan scrubbers
satin over a piece of dimpled foam plastic
jersey over bubble plastic
fine tweed over polyester wadding
stocking stitch in a boucle yarn
stocking stitch in mohair
garter stitch in green plastic string
moss stitch (see below) in random green and brown yarn
basket stitch (see below) in thick wool

For moss stitch, have an even number of stitches, K1 P1 K1 P1 etc. starting every row with K1. Basket stitch is a bit more complicated; choose a number of stitches which is divisible by four and work as follows:

1st row K4 P4 K4 P4 to end.
2nd row P4 K4 etc. (purling the stitches which were knitted in the last row)
Repeat these two rows twice.
7th row P4 K4 etc. (purling the stitches which were purled in the last row)
8th row K4 P4 etc. (knitting the stitches which were purled in the last row)
Repeat rows 7 and 8 twice.

These 12 rows form the pattern; repeat it as many times as required and you will have a chequer board pattern which resembles a woven basket.

When you are satisfied with the pattern of fields, sew them to the backing fabric by hand or using the zig-zag stitch on your machine. Make sure that all the fields are within the tacked line round the mat.

The edges of the fields can be outlined by sewing on green or brown decorative furniture braid, or you can make hedges: cut strips of green towelling, 5 cm wide, and join them together to make the required length. Machine one edge along the edge of the field. Lay four stockings or legs of tights along the towelling, bring the material over them, turn under the raw edge and slipstitch close to the line of machining. Slipstitch the hedges together at the corners of the fields.

Sew small pieces of black or brown Velcro 'loops' in some of the fields. Make trees by cutting circles of green fabric and gathering them around some polyester stuffing. Sew a piece of Velcro 'hooks' over the stitches.

Find six cylindrical threading beads or small cotton reels (about 2 cm long and 2 cm in diameter). Cover them in beige felt and sew them (on their sides) to a beige-coloured field, using strong button thread passed through the hole in the middle of the bead or reel. These are rolls of hay, in case you were wondering!

Finally, turn under the 2 cm border round the mat and back it with another piece of fabric, to neaten the mat and hide all your stitchery.

Hot and Cold

Here are a few ideas:

1. Chia Swee Hong (see above) suggests a pleasant way of experiencing the sensation of cold and warm water. Dip a handtowel into fairly cold or warm water, wring it out, place it in a plastic bag and feel it on hands and feet.
2. Use a Snuggler — a special pack with a soft cover which can be warmed in the microwave and used instead of a hot water bottle.
3. Use heat packs, sold in camping and climbing shops. These gel packs contain a metal disc which, when pressed, causes the gel to give out heat. The packs are reuseable — simmer them in hot water until they are soft again.
4. Place a bag of frozen peas inside a thin cotton cover (to avoid cold burns) and feel the texture and the coldness. The bag can be refrozen and used over and over again, but *don't* eat the peas.
5. A gel eyemask has an interesting texture and is pleasantly cool when it comes out of the fridge.

Air

There are various ways of creating air currents:

- a clean washing-up liquid bottle to puff out air;
- a length of plastic tubing to blow down;
- a fan — battery powered or electric;
- a hairdryer — on cool or warm settings;
- a foot operated pump (from camping shops), used for inflating air beds;
- a balloon pump or bicycle pump;
- a hand blower (Mike Ayres & Co. or Rompa), used for inflating large balls.

Vibration

Vibration seems to be one of the most enjoyable sensations for many people with profound disabilities and I've seen many people who hit their heads rest them instead on a source of vibration or even place it between their teeth. The skull, of course, has its own natural vibrations and resonances.

It is important to remember that the speed of the vibration, and where it is applied, can dramatically affect our enjoyment of it. Some people may prefer a slow rate of vibration, others a much faster; there are people who like vibration on their neck or head, others will hate it. If the person is unable to indicate clearly whether she is enjoying an activity, we must be particularly careful when using vibration and look for the slightest signs of pleasure or discomfort.

There are various items of vibration equipment available commercially, most of which were designed for the general market for health or personal care, rather than for the specialist companies.

1. Massage Tube (Rompa) — a flexible, soft tube which can be held or wrapped round the body. Two speeds of vibration.
2. Vibration Pillow (Rompa) — cushion which vibrates when pressed or leant against.
3. Babyliss Body Toner Plus (from electrical stores) — an electric massager which is as near as possible to having a finger massage. Small knobs move in circles, at two different speeds.
4. Various electric massagers are available, but they tend to be very heavy and tiring to hold for any length of time. Look for the cordless type which are plugged into a base unit for recharging and are much lighter.
5. Massager with Heat (electrical stores, Rompa) — combines vibration with infra-red warmth. Cordless (recharges from the mains-powered base unit) so it is easy to use and lightweight.
6. Battery powered massagers — these are usually intended for facial massage. Availability varies (Clairol have one in their range at the moment) but worth looking out for as they are small and very light.
7. The small lady shavers can be adapted — cover the head completely with PVC tape (so that the moving parts are all hidden). Gather a small circle of towelling or fur fabric over the head. The shavers are light and easy to hold. If you wish, you can add bells or strings of buttons (securely tied round the neck of the shaver) for added interest.
8. Electric toothbrushes (either battery powered or rechargeable) provide vibration and the feel of the brush.
9. Foot Spa (electrical stores) — Clairol was the original make, now there are several. Intended to be used with water, to soothe and massage the feet, they can also be used without water. Place table tennis balls (especially coloured and fluorescent ones), cat balls (with a bell inside), plastic pastry cutters, small plastic dishes and unbreakable Christmas baubles in the dry foot spa and switch on for lots of vibration and noise.
10. Vibrobubble (TFH) — a plastic dome with three pairs of sensors. The dome vibrates when the sensors are touched and there are three different speeds. The Vibrobubble may encourage the use of both hands, and movement of the hands from one pair of sensors to another, but the vibration equipment described above is much cheaper.

Smell

Some people have an acute sense of smell, others have hardly any. Similarly, some people have more interest in and awareness of smells than others. We use our sense of smell to gather information about our surroundings and what is happening, and to discriminate between pleasant and unpleasant smells. Memories are often strongly linked to smells — I only have to smell the musty smell of old buildings and I'm a child playing in the cellar of my grandparents' house! A person's likes and dislikes in terms of smells may be linked to memories of which they may not even be aware.

Smells can also help people to locate where they are — the smell of soap in the bathroom, paint in the artroom, pot pouri in the bedroom, chlorine in the swimming pool, different shops in the high street, and so on.

Some people with profound disabilities don't seem to know how to sniff and if they breathe mainly through their mouths they won't really experience the smells we are offering them. Other people don't know how to sniff gently so pungent odours (whether pleasant or unpleasant) must be well diluted or presented in very small amounts, on a tissue, cotton bud or a smelling strip cut from blotting paper.

It is important to experience a wide range of smells, both nice ones and not so nice ones. Many smells can be introduced into the person's environment, but outings can also be organized with the sense of smell in mind:

1. Toiletries and cosmetics offer a wide range of smells — shampoo, soap, bubble bath, talcum powder, body lotion and handcream, perfume/aftershave, nail varnish and remover.
2. The Body Shop sells a range of products which smell of fruits. The lip balms (e.g. Kiwi) can also be tasted. Their Peppermint Foot Lotion has a wonderful smell and it is cool and refreshing. However, some people with dry, sensitive skin (including me) find that it makes their skin itch — I think it would drive me mad if I couldn't reach my foot to scratch, or tell someone what was wrong!
3. Essential oils (see Aromatherapy section below) offer a range of different types of smell — flowery, fruity, spicy, woody — and pungent ones like tea-tree or eucalyptus.
4. Make your own 'smelly' kit by placing different smells in the plastic pots with close-fitting lids which contain rolls of 35 mm film. Sprinkle liquid smells on cotton wool and place solid smells (herbs, etc.) in a small square of muslin, gathered and tied with cotton, or a short length of Tubegauze finger bandage, with each end tied with cotton. You could also place the smells in clean washing-up liquid bottles, so that the scents can be puffed out.
5. Buy or make your own herb pillows and lavender sachets.
6. Grow pots of fresh herbs on the windowsill.
7. Burn joss sticks.
8. A wide range of pot pouris is available now — use them to identify different rooms.
9. The kitchen offers plenty of interesting smells — onions, herbs, spices, etc. Many tropical fruits (lychees, mangoes, passion-fruit, kiwi fruit) have very strong smells and tastes, and some have textured skins.
10. Visit bakeries, shops which roast and grind coffee beans, flower markets, farms (or city farms), wood mills and engineering workshops.
11. Gardens offer a wide range of smells (see chapter 5).

Taste

Our senses of taste and smell are very closely related and help our full appreciation of the flavour of foods we eat. We can distinguish four different tastes — salt, sweet, bitter and sour. When we are helping someone to discriminate between various tastes, it is best to start with contrasting sweet and savoury and then gradually introduce the range of savoury tastes — sour, salty, bitter, spicy, herbs.

The texture and temperature of food affects our perception of the taste. Try introducing different textures of the same food; for instance banana can be experienced as slices of the fruit, mashed, fried, dried slices, milkshake, instant whip, yogurt, ice lolly.

The taste of food should not be separated from the whole experience of the food — the shape and colour of an orange, the smell as it is peeled, the taste of the flesh or the freshly squeezed juice, for instance.

Work on the sense of taste should be done in conjunction with cooking and eating activities wherever possible, not as an isolated activity. There are so many cookbooks now, with recipes from all over the world, which enable us to try spicy, sweet and sour, and other flavours. Don't forget vegetarian recipes, which often pay more attention to the appearance and texture of the food than meat dishes.

For many people, food is such an overwhelming interest that it can distract them from everything else around. For this reason, I would not work on the sense of taste in a multisensory room, for example.

Aromatherapy and Massage

Aromatherapy is the use of essential oils for therapeutic purposes. The approach is holistic, as the oils affect the physical, mental and emotional state of the person receiving treatment.

The use of essential oils has been recorded in Ancient Egypt, Ancient Greece, during the plagues of the 16th century, and up to the present day. However, modern conventional medicine has been slow to accept the validity of aromatherapy and, in particular, the idea that essential oils placed on the skin can be absorbed into the body and travel to various organs. This has now changed — the skin is not an impermeable layer and drugs for angina, hormone replacement therapy and to combat seasickness can all be administered via a patch on the skin. Many doctors now accept that aromatherapy is a useful and effective form of alternative medicine.

Essential oils are natural plant extracts which are obtained by distillation. Different parts of the plant are used: some oils come from flowers, others from leaves, woody stems, or fruits. The oils are very concentrated and must be used with great care. They are volatile, inflammable, non-greasy and will dissolve in alcohol, water (only partially) and oil. They are synergistic, in other words, combinations of two or three oils are more effective than one on its own.

51

The price of essential oils varies widely. Some oils, such as lavender, are very easy to produce in large quantities and are therefore cheap; others, such as rose, are much more difficult (an enormous quantity of rose petals only yields a small amount of oil) and the oil is extremely expensive.

Good quality, pure oils are available from the suppliers mentioned in the resource list. The oils you can buy in health food shops and those which sell various body preparations are already diluted (which is why they are so much cheaper).

Some oils are stimulating (e.g. lemon), but most are relaxing or calming (e.g. lavender). Some (e.g. geranium) are described as balancing, which means that they regulate the body systems (circulation, lymph system, etc.). Different oils are used to treat various conditions, such as respiratory conditions, digestive problems or skin conditions. This use of oils should only be undertaken by trained aromatherapists who know which oils to use, and when not to use them.

Some oils should not be used if the person has epilepsy. Fennel, hyssop and sage should definitely be avoided; opinions vary about rosemary — some therapists say it is too stimulating but others say that small amounts may be used. If in doubt, consult an aromatherapist about which oils to use, or stick to the really safe ones listed below.

Other oils should not be used in pregnancy (remember that this applies to the person receiving the treatment and the person giving it, if the oils are being used in massage) and some, like lemon and peppermint, may irritate sensitive skins unless used in very small quantities.

Unless you have been on a training course, use ready-made mixtures of oils (see resource list) or the gentle oils:

Relaxing: lavender, camomile, geranium
Refreshing/stimulating: orange, lemon.

Essential oils may be used in various ways:

1. A few drops of a stimulating oil may be placed on a tissue to invigorate the user during a busy day or long journey. A few drops of a relaxing oil may be placed on a pillow to encourage sleep.
2. Essential oils (4-6 drops) may be added to a bath, so that they are inhaled and absorbed through the skin. Oils may also be used in a foot spa.
3. Oils may be vaporized so that they perfume a room and are inhaled by the occupants. Pottery oil burners are widely available in craft shops and from suppliers of oils. Drops of oil (about 10) are placed in a shallow saucer of water which is heated by a nightlight. Electric oil vaporizers are also available (Rompa supply one) and may be preferable in many situations where the presence of a naked flame might cause concern. Also, the pottery burners must not be allowed to run out of water when the flame is lit, as they may crack. Other ways of vaporizing oils include adding them to a bowl of hot water (placed safely out of reach) or to a saucer of water on top of a warm radiator (not an electric one).

4. An air spray can be produced by placing about 30 drops of essential oils in a plant spray and filling with water. Shake well to disperse the oil. The mixture can be left in a brass or ceramic spray, but plastic ones must be rinsed out immediately after use as essential oils react with plastic.
5. Essential oils can be added to a carrier oil and used for massage. This is probably the use that most people immediately think of when aromatherapy is mentioned, but it is important to remember the other uses described above — particularly when massage may not be possible or appropriate.

Massage

Massage can, of course, be carried out using a vegetable oil on its own. However, the addition of essential oils will make the experience much more enjoyable and beneficial. Use three drops of essential oil in every 5 ml of carrier oil. The ideal carrier oil has very little smell and a light consistency. General purpose oils may be purchased from aromatherapy suppliers, but good quality cold-pressed grapeseed or sunflower oils (from health food shops) may also be used. Specialized carrier oils are thicker and more expensive; they are not used on their own, but are added to the basic oil (about 5 per cent of the total volume, usually). Wheatgerm oil is rich in Vitamin E and is a natural anti-oxidant so the massage mixture will keep much longer (up to two or three months). Avocado oil has excellent penetrating properties and therefore helps the essential oils to be absorbed much more quickly.

Aromatherapy massage has so many benefits for people with profound disabilities, as it:

1. encourages relaxation
2. improves circulation, muscle tone and mobility of limbs
3. increases body awareness
4. allows opportunities for choice (different oils, which parts of the body are massaged, when and how)
5. encourages interaction and communication
6. increases tolerance of touch and provides age-appropriate opportunities for personal attention and contact which are not connected with functional touch (toileting, washing, dressing).

Many people are very resistant to touch, perhaps because their experiences of physical contact and handling have not been very pleasant, or because their observation and anticipation skills are not well developed and so physical contact always seems an unexpected and frightening event. It may take a very long time to build up trust to the stage where a simple hand massage is possible, but this is also a process of building a relationship and it is very important.

53

The use of massage raises many issues, such as informed consent, privacy and whether enablers have the training and experience to carry out massage, particularly on people who may be frail.

Unless you have been on a training course, it is wise to concentrate on hand and foot massage and leave body massage to the experts. Massaging hands or feet is a good way of getting to know someone in a fairly non-threatening way and our private space is only being invaded slightly if someone touches our hands or feet.

Although massage should always be carried out in a quiet and relaxed atmosphere, it is possible to do hand and foot massage with other people around, in a variety of settings, whereas privacy is needed if the person is going to strip off for a full body massage. When you are massaging a person's hand or foot, it is possible to position yourself so that you can observe them and check that they are enjoying the experience.

Hand and Foot Massage

The following description of hand and foot massage is taken from 'Aromatherapy and massage for people with learning difficulties' by Helen Sanderson and Jane Harrison with Shirley Price (Hands On Publishing, 1991) and it is included here by kind permission of the authors. I wanted to include this section because it is the clearest description I have found, and with a little study and some practice it should enable you to give a hand or foot massage which is enjoyable for both the receiver and the giver.

Massaging the Hands and Feet

The following instructions serve as a guide for you to follow as you learn to massage. The important thing to remember is that massage is an extension of the natural urge to rub or stroke something better, so it is more important for you to feel your own way and find what feels right and comfortable, than to worry too much about technique. Remember always to explain to the person what you are doing as you begin.

Massaging the Hands

We use our hands so much throughout the day for doing, giving and receiving that it is easy to take them for granted. They are a wonderful part of the body to start massaging. For one thing they are easily accessible and being so sensitive can be an effective way of making contact and affecting the person. Indeed the hands, like the feet, have many reflex points which reflect different parts of the body, so hand massage can affect more than just the health of the hand. As with many types of massage, hand massage can have a variety of effects depending

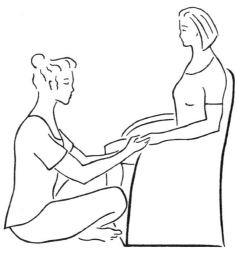

on your intentions. Here are just a few examples of how hand massage has been used for people who have severe learning difficulties:

1. To promote relaxation.
2. To promote body awareness.
3. To relieve stiffness and pain.
4. To break down scar tissue.
5. To improve circulation in the hand.
6. To help the person become accustomed to touch and manipulation of the hand (to improve tolerance of nail cutting for example).
7. To prepare for developing communication, for example hand signing, or through Interactive Massage.
8. To improve relationships and trust.

'Through our arms and hands, we express our most powerful emotions, showing love by embracing, giving, protecting or stroking, hatred or rage through hitting, punching, shaking our fists. An arm and hand massage is thus a marvellously liberating and relaxing experience, especially for those who tend to "bottle up" their feelings' (Clare Maxwell Hudson, 1984).

Some parts of the hand are more sensitive than others. If the person that you are working with is nervous or wary of touch, it is best to start with the least sensitive areas. For example, it may be less threatening for the person if you start on her less dominant hand (i.e. left hand if she is right-handed) and on the back of her hand rather than on her palm. If the aim of your massage is to make the person feel more relaxed and comfortable in herself or with you, then it is worth tuning into the little nuances that will make all the difference.

1. Make sure the person is comfortable, either lying down or sitting up, and that the arm is supported at the elbow (e.g. resting on the arm of the chair), so that the hand can be moved freely without the person having to hold it up for you.

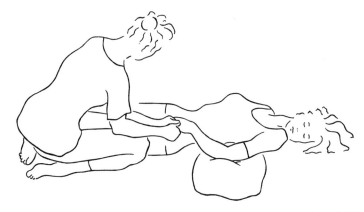

2. Gently but firmly make some contact with the person's hand. Hold the whole hand sandwiched between your own for a few seconds or just lay one hand over the person's wrist.

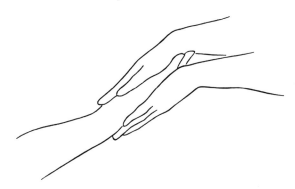

3. Lift the person's hand and holding it firmly underneath with your fingers, slowly and firmly draw the heels of both your hands from the middle of the person's hand outwards. Stop when the heels of your hands are at the edge of the person's hand. Do this several times to open and stretch it.

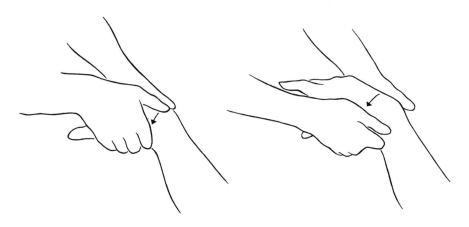

4. Now use your thumbs to work in small circles over the whole area of the back of the hand, up between the bones of the hand and around the bones of the wrist.

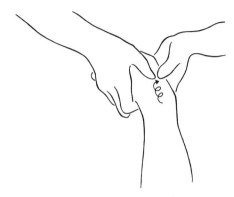

5. Turn the person's hand palm up and supporting the back of the hand this time with your fingers, massage with your thumbs in small clockwise movements over the whole palm, working all the muscles and joints and opening up the hand.
6. Now move onto the fingers. Hold the person's hand with one of yours and wrapping your whole hand or thumb and forefinger round the person's thumb, gently slide your fingers up from the base to the tip of the thumb. Pull a little as you go and twist your hand from side to side as you would opening a bottle with a corkscrew. Don't pull too hard. It is good to give the joints a gentle stretch but not to force them to crack. Do each finger in the same way.

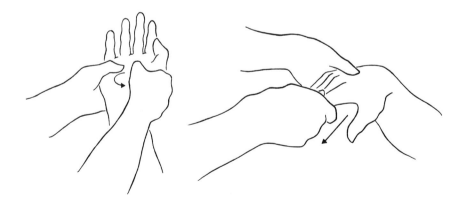

7. Gently rotate each finger. If the person finds it difficult to relax or if she wants to be helpful she may do the movement for you. If you want to help her to relax and to 'let go', slow your movement or reverse the direction.

57

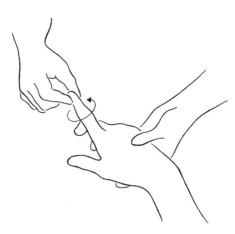

8. End by holding the person's whole hand again between both of yours. Lay it back down gently. Repeat with the other hand. It is always nice if you have time to massage both hands or both feet. You will certainly notice the difference in tension and a feeling of imbalance if you have had only one hand massaged.

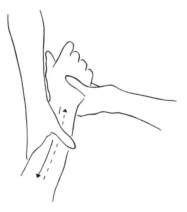

9. If you want to massage the forearm as well to stimulate the circulation down to the hand, hold the hand with one of yours. With the other hand hold the arm with your fingers together down one side and your thumb the other and using long smooth strokes work firmly up the arm drawing the hand lightly down each time to start again.

Massaging the Feet

Reflexology is based on the principle that there are points or areas of the feet and hands that correspond to each part of the body. By rubbing and working on these points reflexologists can improve the overall health of a person. Massaging the foot inevitably touches many of these points and a good foot massage can do much to reduce overall tension. Many of us live 'up in our heads', thinking and worrying, detached from our feet and legs. Headaches and cold feet are a clear sign that the body is out of balance. Foot massage can draw the attention down, thus helping to restore balance. Notice how quickly the feet warm up whilst massaging them.

Although foot massage will not correct deformities such as contractures it can improve the overall condition, circulation and flexibility of the foot. For people who are nervous about having their toe-nails cut or seeing the chiropodist, foot massage is a pleasant way to help the person become accustomed to having her feet handled. For some individuals, their only experience of their feet being touched may be having shoes and socks put on them. If a person has poor circulation, her awareness of her feet may be diminished. Using massage and essential oils, after using a foot spa and drying the feet with a warm fluffy towel, the feet may be appreciated in a different way. The strokes for the feet are very similar to those for the hand. You may find that a carrier lotion with added essential oils gives a smoother movement than a carrier oil.

1. Make sure the person is comfortable, either sitting up or, preferably, lying down. Make sure that the person can relax her foot and does not have to hold it up for you. Prop it up on a cushion or on your own leg.

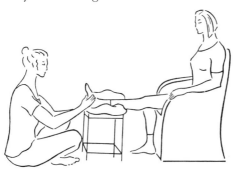

2. Make some contact. Lay one hand over the person's foot or sandwich the foot between your hands.

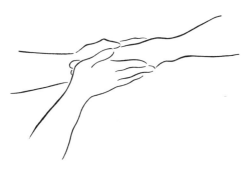

3. Holding the foot between the hands stroke firmly up the foot several times from the toes to the heel and ankle.

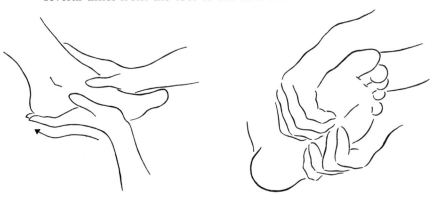

4. Then hold it firmly underneath with your fingers and use the heels of your hands to open and stretch the top of the foot from the middle outwards.

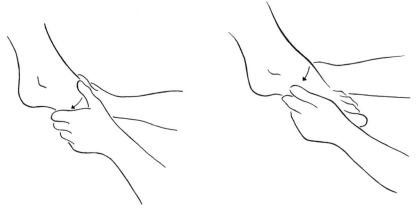

5. Holding the foot with your fingers, go over the top of the foot with your thumbs working in small circular movements. Make sure you cover the whole area slowly and thoroughly.

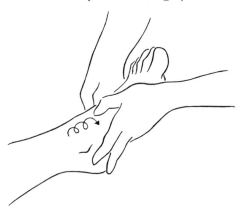

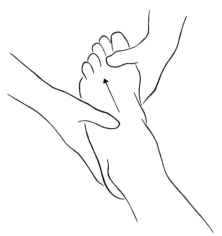

6. Draw your thumb up once along each valley between the tendons that run from the ankle to the toes.
7. Next work over the sole of the foot using your thumbs in the same way. You may find some hard crystal-like areas. They may be a little tender to work on but are an indication that that particular reflex is blocked. Sometimes these blocks may be easily alleviated but don't overwork points that are very tender. They may reflect quite a chronic area of ill-health, better left to a qualified reflexologist. Again, cover the whole area.
8. When you reach the heel, gently lift it up and work all round the heel with your thumbs and fingertips.

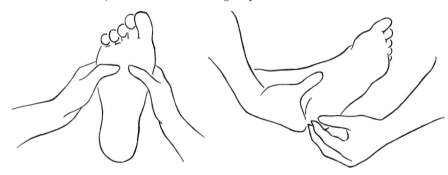

9. Lay the foot down and circle the ankle bone itself on either side of the ankle. Circle it several times with your fingertips. Go gently if this is tender for the person.

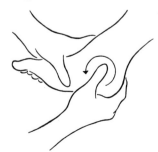

61

10. Now on to the toes. As with the fingers, slide your wrapped hand or finger and thumb from the base to the tip of each one pulling gently as you go.
11. Gently rotate each toe holding it at the tip. Rotation of the big toe is excellent for relieving head tension and headaches.
12. End by holding the whole foot again, sandwiched between your hands.
13. Repeat these strokes on the other foot.

Interactive Massage (Sanderson, Harrison and Price, 1991)

The authors of 'Aromatherapy and massage for people with learning difficulties' also describe two other ways of using aromatherapy: Interactive Massage and Multisensory Massage.

In their book 'Deaf-Blind Infants and Children: A Developmental Guide' (1982), McInnes and Treffry describe the Interactive Sequence. This is a series of responses which we will usually observe when we introduce a new stimulus (an activity or a piece of equipment) to a person who has a dual sensory impairment. The same responses are often observed in people with profound disabilities, particularly if they have been used to an environment which offers few exciting or new experiences.

The stages of the Interactive Sequence are:

1. Resists
2. Tolerates
3. Co-operates passively
4. Enjoys
5. Responds co-operatively
6. Leads
7. Imitates
8. Initiates

In massage, stages one to four are passive — the person moves gradually from resisting to enjoying the massage, but does not take an active part. Stages five to eight are interactive massage, in which the person begins to respond (by offering her hand, for example), leads the activity (by offering the other hand, when one is finished), imitates (by copying the strokes on her hand, or by massaging the enabler's hand) and finally initiates the activity (finding the oil and taking it to the enabler, or leading her to the room where massage usually takes place).

Passive massage may be relaxing or invigorating, but it does not expect any response from the person receiving it. Interactive massage aims to increase communication and interaction by encouraging the person to respond to the activity and participate in it.

Multisensory Massage (Sanderson, Harrison and Price, 1991)

An aromatherapy massage can be a multisensory experience in itself: the smell of the oils, the touch and movement of the massage, the sound of relaxing music. Sensory stimulation can be increased through multisensory massage. This is the use of different massage tools, as well as essential oils, to stimulate the senses. The massage may be passive or interactive, depending on the person and their needs.

Different massage tools — footsie roller, handle roller, six ball massage roller, body buddy (all from The Body Shop) can be used on different parts of the body. It is important to remember that we may not like a particular sensation but we can say so, and make sure that we don't have to experience it. We must be sensitive to whether the person is enjoying an activity or not. Electric massagers and other items which vibrate, such as the Massage Tube (Rompa) or a Foot Spa, seem to be very popular with many people, particularly if they have sensory impairments.

Movement

A person who has had few opportunities to experience large movements — swinging, rolling, bouncing, stretching, rocking, moving in water — is unlikely to have a well-developed sense of her own body and limbs, the relationship between her body and her surroundings, or awareness of weight, centre of gravity, balance and posture. A movement programme can help to develop body awareness and motor skills. For some people the programme will be active, for others it will be more passive as the enablers support them and move their bodies and limbs through the activities.

One of the most influential people in movement work was Veronica Sherborne, who applied Rudolf Laban's theories of human movement to the needs of children, with and without disabilities. She believed that movement experiences are fundamental to the development of all children and that the input of movement experiences has to be more concentrated and continuous for children with disabilities. Her philosophy applies equally to adults with severe and profound disabilities and many of the people she taught now work in adult services. Further information on resources and training courses is given in chapter 11.

Any movement session should always start with gentle warming up exercises. Mats, bean-bag seats, floor cushions or duvets can be used to make the person comfortable. If necessary you can provide physical support by sitting with your legs on either side of the person and her body leaning against yours. If the person is heavy, or you are going to be in this position for long, you will also need support — sit with your back against a wall or a solid piece of furniture. In this position you can do various rocking, stretching and other movement activities to music.

Some ideas for movement activities:

63

1. Lie the person on a blanket on a smooth floor. Pull them around the floor, varying the speed, turning corners, gently swaying from side to side.
2. Use a parachute (see chapter 8) for gentle stretching movements — raising the parachute expands the rib cage and helps breathing exercises.
3. Use a parachute for dancing to lively folk music — move round in a circle, into the centre and out, stay still and pass the parachute round.
4. Dye lengths of muslin (available from education catalogues at a reasonable price) in various colours and use them for wafting and shaking, or gently pulling over people lying on mats.
5. Machine several silky headscarves together to form a large square or rectangle and use them in place of the muslin (above).
6. The slightest movement of an arm or hand is magnified if the person is holding a fan (paper, feather or cane — from oriental shops), a ribbon streamer (from education catalogues), a chiffon or silky scarf, or a parasol.
7. Keep a balloon in the air by patting, blowing or kicking it.
8. Pass a ball or quoit around the group; stretch high or bend low to pass it through a hoop.
9. Roll a large ball around or across a circle of people.
10. 'Sensory-Motor Integration Activities' (Winslow Press) is a ringbinder full of movement ideas which can be used with individuals or groups.
11. 'Activity Programmes for Body Awareness, Contact and Communication' (Winslow Press) is an activity programme designed to improve sensory, perceptual and motor skills. The specially-composed music is attractive and suitable for adults.

Yoga

There is increasing interest in the use of yoga with people with disabilities. Yoga has both physical benefits (improved posture and increased suppleness) and mental benefits (increased self-confidence and awareness, calmness and a decrease in tension). If you wish to introduce yoga to people with profound disabilities, you will need to find a qualified teacher with some experience in this field or to encourage a teacher and a physiotherapist to work together to explore the possibilities.

There are various books and training courses on yoga for people with disabilities (see chapter 11).

Electronic Games

She writes:Many of the electronic games which are so popular at the moment offer a lot of stimulation, with bright lights and loud noises. When choosing games, it is important to check the brightness and loudness of the effects. If the game offers various skill levels, are the first levels simple enough? Can you get some of the light and sound effects even if you cannot play the game properly? Most games come with instruction booklets — take a photocopy and keep it in a safe place, ready for when the booklet gets lost!

One of the best games is the Tandy Computer Arcade (there are Tandy shops in many large towns). This has twelve large buttons which light up. The coloured lights are fairly bright (particularly in a darkened room) and the electronic notes are loud. There are twelve games altogether; some of them are complicated and skilful but there are simple ones as well. Switching the machine on causes each button to light up and play its note in sequence. In the 'Organ' game, each button operates when pressed. 'Songwriter' memorizes the notes you play (up to 47 notes) and then plays them back to you, over and over again. In 'Tag-It' one button flashes at a time, pressing that button quickly enough produces a beep.

The problem with most electronic games is that they don't like getting wet. Electronic parts and keyboards can be covered with clingfilm to protect them from dribbling. Check the clingfilm regularly to make sure that it is not coming off, as it could be a choking or suffocation hazard.

'Gimmicky' Things

Many of the most successful items for sensory stimulation are the gimmicky things which are all the rage one moment and disappear the next. They are the sort of things you find in bargain stores, on market stalls, at the seaside or fairgrounds. Many wonderful items have come and gone, and the items described below may well have disappeared by the time this book is published. The important thing is to keep your eyes open all the time for items which will be useful in a sensory bank, and when you see them — buy them!

These are some of the things we have been enjoying:

1. Animal Quackers — small animal head (duck, pig, frog) on a strap. They are sold for children to wear on their ankles and the slightest movement produces a very realistic animal noise. They must contain some kind of tilt switch, yet they sell at £1.99 — a mercury tilt switch from a specialist supplier would cost considerably more!
2. Breaking Glass Ball (or Rock) — these soft foam balls or 'rocks' make a very realistic sound of broken glass when hit or dropped.
3. Groan Tube — plastic tube, in fluorescent colours, which makes a groaning noise when you turn it over.
4. Laughing Mirror/Laughter Bag — peals of crazy laughter when you pick the mirror up or squeeze the bag.
5. Pin Sculpture — thousands of stainless steel pins (without points) which take the impression of any three-dimensional firm object. Guess what made the impression, compare faces or hands. Interesting texture and light/shade effects.

6. Rainbow Lite-Up — a plastic disc lights up and rolls along two metal prongs; wonderful effect in a darkened room.
7. Singing Sponge — bath sponge with a small metal button inside which, when pressed, plays a tune.

Some suppliers of this type of equipment are listed in chapter 11, but your best bet is to look in joke shops, executive toy sections of department stores, cut-price shops, and so on.

5

Multisensory Environments

Multisensory Rooms

This section looks at various types of multisensory rooms and the ways in which they are used. There has been a tremendous upsurge of interest in the concept in recent years and there is a certain element of 'jumping on the bandwagon' by both service providers and commercial firms. However, there is no doubt that multisensory rooms and the equipment they contain can offer a wealth of new experiences for people with profound disabilities.

The original multisensory room was developed in Holland in a residential unit for people with learning disabilities. The staff created '*Snoezelen*' to provide a leisure facility which offered gentle stimulation and relaxation, and an opportunity for enablers and clients to share experiences and communicate with each other. Above all, it was an environment in which there was no pressure to achieve, to learn skills, or to live up to other people's expectations.

I believe it is important to remember these original aims, in view of the developments which we are witnessing now. Multisensory rooms are intended to be experienced by clients and enablers together; unfortunately many of the rooms are used as dumping grounds, in the hope that people will enjoy the lights, sounds, etc. while their enablers get on with 'more important things'. The development of computerized control systems, which operate all the effects, makes it even more tempting to believe that the presence of enablers is not necessary.

Snoezelen was developed to provide leisure and pleasure, not as a venue for assessment and skills training. The development of interactive environments which seek, quite properly, to give people control over their leisure environment has encouraged therapists to hijack multisensory rooms for assessment and treatment purposes. I realize that, when money is tight, there is a temptation to demonstrate that an expensive installation can be used for a variety of purposes, including important things like education and therapy. When will people accept that appropriate leisure use is sufficient justification alone?

Since *Snoezelen* was introduced into the United Kingdom by Rompa (who hold the registered trademark), many firms have developed their own ranges of multisensory equipment. Most of the companies also offer a design and installation service. There are wide variations in prices and in the amount of after-sales support and servicing you can expect, so it is essential to shop around. Compare prices for various components, ask plenty of questions about the design package and ask to visit some installations so that you can get ideas for your room and, more importantly, talk to these previous customers to see if they were satisfied with the service they received.

Companies which supply multisensory equipment are listed in chapter 11, together with details of training courses, books and videos.

A multisensory room is usually painted white, to show up the lighting effects, and has no natural light. It is possible to buy foam mattresses (covered with white PVC) to cover the floor but some people prefer to have white vinyl floor covering with specific sitting/lying areas dotted around the room. Both options have good and bad points. The mattresses are not easy to walk on and enablers can hurt their backs when they are trying to lift someone, but people can sit or lie in comfort wherever they like in the room. A hard floor is easier for walking or manoevring a wheelchair, but there is less freedom of choice in the room.

Various items are available for sitting or lying:

1. Bean bags covered with white PVC — although these are, quite rightly, frowned on by physiotherapists for long-term use they can be useful in the multisensory room for positioning people so that they are comfortable and can see the effects.
2. Water or air mattresses are popular, but they take up a lot of room.
3. Leaf Chair (Mike Ayres & Co., TFH) — this is a hanging chair which is very comfortable and relaxing. It can be difficult to lift heavy people into the chair and plenty of space is needed so that people are not too close to the gentle swinging movement of the chair.

There are some pieces of equipment which most people choose to have in their multisensory room:

1. Solar Projector with effect wheels and a rotator. The effect wheels offer various patterns, colours or pictures (clouds, balloons, flowers, spaceships, etc.) which move around the room. Effect cassettes are also available; these give more stimulating visual effects, with brightly coloured geometric patterns. Various other accessories for the projector are available. The projector must be positioned out of reach of people using the room, to avoid damage or injury, but where it can be reached conveniently by enablers to change the effect wheels.

   Project the image onto the walls, a projection tent (from Kirton Litework), the floor or the ceiling (a deflector mirror fitted to the projector will make this easier). Hang lengths of net curtain in the beam of the projector — this is a useful way of bringing the image closer to someone. If you hang two pieces of net curtain about 10 cm apart, you will get an interesting double image.
2. Bubble Tube — this is a plastic column, filled with water. The column is

lit from below and the colours change gradually, while streams of bubbles rise up the tube. As well as the visual effect, there is the noise of the motor and pump and the tube vibrates slightly. The impact of the light, colours and bubbles can be increased by placing a curved acrylic mirror behind the tube. A similar effect can be achieved by sticking pieces of diffraction foil or survival blanket to the wall. The bubble tube produces a lot of light, which can overshadow other light effects in a small room — try switching it off occasionally, so that other pieces of equipment can be enjoyed.

3. Mirror Ball — the ball rotates and, with a spotlight shining on it, reflects points of light around the room. Colour filters for the pinspot are available, but I prefer white light — there are enough coloured lights in the room. The mirror ball can be fixed to the ceiling; there is also a portable model on a stand but I feel this is just one more thing to keep an eye on, in case it gets knocked over. I prefer the Domed Half Mirror Ball (from Environmental Electrical Services). It is expensive, but it is so much more versatile than a mirror ball fixed to the ceiling. The Dome is on the floor, so people can lie beside it, see the reflections, hear the motor and touch the Perspex cover. Also, you can move the Dome into other rooms and place it in the sunshine to get beautiful 'Jack-a-Dandies' shining around the room.

4. Sideglow Fibre Optic Spray — this is a spray of plastic-covered strands which shine along their length. The colours change gradually, with a shimmering effect, and the strands can be handled or spread over people.

5. Rope Light — this is a long plastic tube containing coloured lights which flash and appear to travel along the tube. The rate of flashing can be adjusted. One of the cheapest rope lights is available from Innovations. It is very effective but the control unit is rather fragile and it is not always easy to adjust the speed. For about the same price, Messenger and Clark sell a rope light which is very attractive and sturdy and the speed can be easily adjusted from zero (one colour permanently lit) to very rapid.

6. Cassette recorder and tapes — a wide range of relaxing music and natural sound recordings is available (see chapter 11 for details) and will add a great deal to the enjoyment of the multisensory room. It is useful to have a machine with twin decks and a pause facility, so that you can play cassettes with the minimum of interruption.

7. Many companies supply pieces of equipment which blow smells into the room. I don't think these are very satisfactory, or represent value for money, and I prefer to introduce smells in a 'low tech' way. Essential oils can be vaporized or diluted in water and sprayed around the room. Don't get carried away — use the oils sparingly, otherwise people may end up feeling rather overwhelmed and 'headachey'.

Tactile stimulation can be introduced into the room by making wall-mounted texture boards. Several companies supply these, but I don't see the point of paying someone to make something that you can make more easily.

Doing it yourself not only saves money but enables you to use the sort of textures you want.

One of the best pieces of equipment I have seen in a multisensory room was a brightly-lit aquarium mounted in the wall at floor level, so that people could lie on a mattress beside it. Who needs complicated machinery when you have beautifully coloured fish swimming backwards and forwards?

There are so many DIY ideas you can use in the multisensory room (many of the examples in chapter 4, for instance) — here are some ideas which were given to me by Julie Redwood from Douglas House in Bournemouth:

1. Bunches and swags of fluorescent netting on the ceiling and walls.
2. Chunks of polystyrene or polystyrene packing shapes threaded on string and hung from the ceiling — they absorb the light and colours from the Solar projector.
3. Survival blanket attached to the wall, with strips of irridescent cellophane (from some art shops and education catalogues) attached to the blanket.
4. Sheets of pegboard attached to the walls with pieces of sheepskin, foam plastic and pan scourers glued on. Feathers, pine-cones and shells are tied on (through the holes in the pegboard) and strands of the metal foil from an old glitter pompom are poked through the holes (use a crochet hook to pull them through). A piece of strong sailcloth (very scrunchy) is also attached.
5. Door screens are made by attaching lengths of strong tinsel (the thick, expensive kind) or strings of bells and beads to pieces of dowel or broom handle which are attached above the door.

Many other pieces of commercial equipment are available, and there are new developments all the time. It is important to be selective — consider what the equipment actually offers, does it represent value for money, does it offer a different type of sensory stimulation from your existing equipment (or is it just a variation on a theme)? Above all, ask yourself if you want the piece of equipment because it will be enjoyed by your clients, or because it appeals to you!

Many companies are becoming increasingly interested in the design of interactive equipment, which enables the user to control the visual or other effects by means of switches or by making sounds.

A multisensory room can be a very large installation, or a small room. It is important to remember that you can start in a very small way, with two or three pieces of equipment, and develop the room slowly — you don't have to buy in the whole design package unless you want to and can afford it.

Our own multisensory room at Planet's resource centre aims to demonstrate what can be done in a small space, on a limited budget. The room was the size of a small bedroom, with two windows, patterned wallpaper and a dark carpet. We painted over the wallpaper with white emulsion and covered the windows with 'blackout' fabric. This is a white, very dense fabric used for lining curtains to exclude the light (available from suppliers of curtain fabrics). The material was cut to the size of the window frame and pieces of Velcro 'loops' were machined at intervals along each edge. Corresponding pieces of self-adhesive Velcro 'hooks' were stuck round the window frame.

The room had heating pipes running round two sides, at floor level. These were boxed in with wood (painted white), which made a sturdy low seat. This has proved ideal for people who are not yet relaxed enough to sit or lie on the floor. Most of the floor was covered by a king-size duvet with a plain cover made from two white sheets. This is easy to walk on but soft and warm to lie on. The rest of the floor is covered by a white polyester fleece underblanket. There are also several pillows with white pillowcases, which are useful for making people comfortable.

Wooden battens are fixed round the walls at picture rail height, so that we can easily stretch lengths of curtain wire across the room to suspend strips of net curtain and a bird mobile. Reflex panels (from Kirton Litework or Rompa) are stuck to the walls and the inside of the door (at low level). These reflect the lights from their different patterns.

A projection tent (from Kirton Litework) provides a smaller environment within the room, with battery powered Christmas-tree lights attached round the opening (using self-adhesive Velcro). A small, white trolley, half hidden behind the tent, holds the cassette recorder and tapes, plus an electric diffuser for essential oils.

When we first started the room, this was all we had — plus a ropelight and a half mirror dome (see above). Until we could have a spotlight fixed in position, a small penlight produced very satisfactory lights around the room.

Later, when we had more money, we added a bubble tube with a curved mirror behind it, a large acrylic mirror on one wall, a fibre optic sideglow spray and a Solar projector with various effect wheels. The projector stands on a wall-mounted television shelf, and a deflector mirror enables us to move the image around the room — to shine on the floor, the ceiling or the projection tent. A white beanbag provides alternative seating.

In total we have spent about £2 000 on the room — a fraction of the amount many people spend.

Most multisensory rooms are white, but some people use a totally black room. These are fine for specific light stimulation work and the use of UV light sources (see chapter 4), but they can be very oppressive and claustrophobic for a leisure facility. If space is limited and you want a black room and a white room, try this idea: paint the walls black, fix plastic covered washing line along the top of each wall and hang up white fabric or old sheets using shower curtain rings. These white curtains can be drawn across the walls when required.

Other small, temporary multisensory environments can be created using the projection tent, or by creating a tent with a parachute. Most parachutes are brightly coloured and will not be very suitable for projecting coloured lights. Flying Objects (see chapter 11) sell lovely soft, silky parachutes in one pale colour (e.g. green). There is a loop in the centre of the parachute, which can be used to hang it from a beam or a hook. The tent shape can be formed by tying string at intervals round the edge of the parachute and attaching it to convenient anchorage points or pieces of furniture. The effect wheels of the Solar projector, and other light sources, will show up well on the pale colour. You can also blow bubbles under the canopy and introduce textures, smells and so on. Place an electric fan under the parachute tent, with strips of fabric tied to the grille of the fan. If you place drops of essential oils on the fabric, you will get scent as well as colour and movement.

Objects can be hung from the parachute, but don't use safety pins, which may tear the fabric if objects are pulled. Either bunch a small piece of the parachute and tie string firmly round it (the creases will come out later) or machine Velcro pieces (use 'loops' — 'hooks' may scratch people when the parachute is being used for games).

Theme Work

Theme work can make new experiences more understandable, because they occur within a context, and it can certainly help enablers. Having a theme may trigger ideas for activities and props, help to keep the momentum going and make everyone feel that they know what's going on and what's expected of them.

Some themed packages are available, for instance the music and drama packs from The Consortium:

1. Galaxies is a multisensory event based on space travel. The pack consists of colour slides, an audio cassette with the story, songs and sound effects and a handbook which gives the words for the songs and describes the props which need to be made.
2. Seaside consists of two cassettes of songs (plus instrumental versions), suggested scripts and ideas for activities using readily available equipment.

These packs can be combined with other equipment you may have. For instance, Galaxies could be used in a multisensory room with a bubble tube as the spacecraft's engines, and the space effect wheel on the Solar projector.

You can make up your own themes based on objects (e.g. trees), places (e.g. gardens) or events (e.g. holidays, Christmas). Leon Charman, from the RNIB's Sunshine House School in Northwood, told me about some theme work he organized. The theme was rainbows; each week they concentrated on a particular colour of the rainbow and all the activities, food, decorations, clothes were linked to that colour. On the eighth week, all the colours came together in the rainbow.

Whatever the theme, try to build in as many relevant sensory experiences as possible and involve everyone in planning the materials, activities, music, and so on.

Outdoors

The biggest and best multisensory environment ever! Think of all the experiences the outdoors can offer — whether you live in the country or in a town.

The feel of soft drizzle, wind, or snow; the sound of wind or heavy rain; the warmth of the sun, the cold wetness of a snowflake. Listen to the wind howling round buildings or sighing in the branches of a tree, the sound of water running down an outside drain or in a stream.

Explore the shape and texture of twigs, bark, pine cones, shiny conkers in velvety cases. Watch the sun sparkling on water, grasses moving in the breeze, autumn leaves blowing into drifts.

Go pond dipping, or play Poohsticks (see chapter 8). Visit accessible nature reserves and bird sanctuaries, parks and gardens, city farms. Don't forget the unpleasant sounds and smells of town and country life, as well as the nice ones!

Sensory Gardens

Every garden, however small or large, is a multisensory experience but with a little thought and planning the possibilities can be extended and made more accessible.

Think about the structure of the garden:

1. Raised flower-beds will bring the plants closer to people and enable them to help with the gardening chores. They will also enable you to grow plants which would not tolerate your soil conditions, because you can fill the bed with the correct type of soil.
2. Different path surfaces will add interest and help visually impaired people to locate where they are in the garden. Gravel looks and sounds attractive but may be difficult for wheelchair users. Concrete setts, in cement, make an interesting texture which is much easier to walk on than cobbles. Different colours and shapes of paving stones can be used. If herbs like thyme and camomile are allowed to spill over the edges of paths, they will release their scent when they are brushed against. The same effect can be achieved by planting herbs in the gaps between crazy paving but if the plants get too big, they may trip people up.
3. Water always adds another dimension in a garden, providing movement, reflections and sound. A flat bridge can be constructed over a stream or pond, using railway sleepers or sturdy planks and wooden railings. This will enable people to sit or stand and look down into the water, drop pebbles in (provided there are no fish to frighten) and get a different view of the garden. Stop people slipping on the wooden planks by fixing chicken wire over the surface with wire staples.

   If you are worried about the possible dangers of a pond, a fountain running over pebbles or an old millstone will be an attractive addition to the garden.

4. A pergola, an arch or a simple pole up which climbing plants can be trained, will bring the sight and smell of the flowers closer to people.
5. Provide garden seats at various points, so that people can sit and enjoy the garden. A hammock would be a lovely change from a conventional seat. If there are no suitable trees available, set two Metapost metal sockets in concrete, insert two fenceposts with sturdy hooks bolted into them, and suspend the hammock from these.

Sounds

1. Water — stream, waterfall or fountain.
2. Hang windchimes from trees or a washing line (the birds will soon get used to them).
3. Plant bamboo and other ornamental grasses which will rustle in the wind.
4. Encourage birds into the garden by installing a bird table, hanging feeders and nesting boxes in the trees. Plant shrubs with winter berries (such as Cotoneaster and Pyrocanthus); grow sunflowers (which are easy and spectacular) and leave the seedheads for the birds. Most birds are attracted by red and yellow flowers (as anyone who has planted yellow crocuses will know!)
5. Attract bees and butterflies by planting blue-flowered plants (especially Ceanothus, Buddleia and lavenders), blossom trees and wild flower seed mixtures.

Touch

1. Many plants can be touched without damaging them — some have furry leaves or ones with interesting shapes. Different shapes and sizes of bulbs can be explored and planted. Remember that some plants contain irritants which may affect some people — primulas, honeysuckle, tomato plants and hyacinth bulbs, for instance.
2. Plant trees with different textured bark — rough, smooth, the white papery bark of silver birch. The weeping willow provides a curtain of twigs and leaves to be explored and pushed through.
3. Introduce sculptures and other garden ornaments and position them where they can be handled.

Taste

1. A wide range of vegetables, orchard fruits and soft fruits can be grown — both those which can be eaten immediately and those which are

taken indoors to prepare and cook. Many vegetables are very attractive when they are growing, and some of the more unusual ones (such as sweetcorn or globe artichokes) are particularly interesting.

2. The new Ballerina apple trees bring the blossom and fruit nearer to people, and take up less space.

Shape and Colour

1. Create different shapes in the garden by the way you use paths and walls, but also in the planting. Conifers offer several different shapes — conical, rounded, low growing — as do other trees and shrubs. Contrast spiky foliage or single stems, like red-hot pokers, against a softer background.
2. Plant flowering plants in blocks of a single colour, so that they show up clearly. Place hanging baskets or tubs containing flowers of one colour against a white painted wall.

Scent

So many plants have attractive or unusual scents that it can be hard to know where to begin. Some varieties of a particular species may smell stronger than others — visit garden centres, specialist nurseries, or flower shows and take notes on the ones you like best.

Try to choose a range of plants which will give a succession of smells throughout the year, and separate out the scents by planting them in different parts of the garden or by positioning a winter scenting plant next to a summer one. In this way each scent can be enjoyed individually, rather than as a confusing mixture, and different parts of the garden can be identified. Planting in areas sheltered by bushes or walls will help the scent to hang in the air, rather than being blown away on the breeze. Training plants such as wisteria, jasmine and honeysuckle over arches will help to surround the person with scent.

Once you have your scented plants, make sure that people have opportunities to enjoy them. Witch-hazel and viburnum have a strong perfume in winter, so wrap up warmly and go and smell them! Night scented stocks, tobacco plants, sweet rocket and evening primrose are beautiful at dusk — plant them under living-room and bedroom windows but also make opportunities for people to be outside to smell the plants and watch the moths which are attracted to these plants, as well as to outside lights and torches.

Most flowering plants have scents which have been used or imitated by the perfume industry, but some plants have much more unusual smells — lemon balm, bergamot (smells of orange), fennel (aniseed), iris (some varieties smell of vanilla or chocolate), curry plant, and so on. Then there are the herbs like basil, bay, chives, marjoram, rosemary, sage, thyme and the mints which have various scents — apple, eau de cologne, ginger, peppermint, pineapple. All the mints are very invasive and are best grown in large pots or tubs to keep them under control and the scents separate.

Sources of advice on designing sensory gardens are listed in chapter 11. Remember that some of the advice may be intended for gardens which are designed specifically for people with visual impairment — you may need to be more careful about which plants are poisonous.

6

Creating

This chapter considers various creative activities; it is not the appropriate place for a discussion of creativity — other authors do this far better than I ever could (and their books are listed in chapter 11) — but I have tried to gather together some practical ideas which may be of interest.

As with any new experience, we must be sensitive when offering these materials — people need time to understand what is happening, explanations, opportunities to explore the new sensation at their own pace, and the chance to say 'No' if they don't like it. They may be resistant to new textures, anxious about getting wet or dirty, or need time to decide if they like the activity. Whilst I believe that 'No' should be respected, this does not mean that we never offer the activity again — a different day (or time of day) or a different enabler may produce a different response.

It is important to think about the new experience we are offering and how it will feel to the recipient. I once visited a unit where an enabler expressed surprise that a client reacted badly when his feet were placed in cold finger paint. He couldn't see what was about to happen, he probably would not have been able to understand a verbal explanation (if one had been given, which it was not), one moment his feet were covered in warm woolly socks and the next they were bare and plunged into something cold and wet. How would you feel?

. . . A Mess!

Messy play is a very important activity for children, offering sensory stimulation, opportunities to explore natural materials and an activity which has few rules (apart from safety considerations) about the 'right' or 'wrong' way to use the materials. As adults, we continue to have opportunities for messy play — gardening, washing the car, DIY activities (e.g. mixing concrete, using putty), cooking (e.g. making bread or pastry), washing up, and so on.

It is important for people with profound disabilities to have such opportunities but enablers often have concerns about the appropriateness of the activities offered. Many feel that playing with sand should only happen on the beach. I agree, in principle, but as most people's visits to a sandy beach are rather limited we have to find other ways of providing similar experiences. Sand doesn't have to be in a childish sandpit or tray, it can be in a large washing-up bowl or a Tidy Sheet (from Lakeland Plastics) for example.

Sand or water activities can form part of theme work on the seaside or holidays, rather than an activity on their own. Water and bubble activities can be part of a daily living skill, like washing up or bathing, but allow time for the fun as well as the chore!

Sand

Sand is a very versatile material, having totally different properties when it is dry, damp or wet. Dry sand feels cool, silky and gentle as it runs through your fingers; it can be used with sieves and funnels and you can bury objects and find them again.

Damp sand can be moulded and sculpted into shapes and objects can be pressed into the surface to leave impressions. Wet sand forms a 'slurry' which can be dribbled through your hands to form weird and wonderful shapes. Adding washing-up liquid and water to sand creates an interesting texture, but only use a small quantity of sand as it will never recover from this treatment!

Cold, wet sand can feel rather unpleasant — try using hot water which, when mixed with the sand, will be pleasantly warm.

Make sure that you buy the right sort of sand. Silver sand is fine for dry use, but it won't dampen properly. Ask a builders' merchant for 'washed playgroup sand' or buy it from educational catalogues.

Water

Water can be contained in a sink, bath, bowl or commercial water tray. Provide a variety of objects (some which will float and others which will sink) including colanders, sieves and funnels. Sponges and lengths of plastic tubing will add to the fun, and the mess!

Add food colouring, food essences (to create different smells) and washing-up liquid for added interest and sensory stimulation. If you have a transparent water tray, you can shine torches and other coloured lights through the water, from below or the sides.

A Foot Spa (Clairol and other makes) is an ideal individual water tray, as it keeps the water warm and has vibration as well. Colour the water with food colourings and shine a bright light on the surface. Add essential oils (or use food essences if the person may drink the water). Always use the foot spa with a residual current circuit breaker, for safety.

Bubbles

Bubbles fascinate most people, both those who are producing them and those who watch. Their irridescent colours, the way they move in the air, and the little splash when they burst are all part of the attraction. Don't allow bubbles to burst in people's eyes (definitely not a pleasant sensory experience!) but bursting them on bare arms or legs is fun.

The basic recipe for bubble mixture is:

1/4 cup of good quality washing-up liquid or baby bubblebath
1 cup water
Glycerine (from chemists or cake-decorating shops)

The glycerine makes the bubbles stronger and more colourful. Adding Gelozone (a thickening agent, available from health food shops) will make the bubbles even stronger.

There are various commercial bubble kits available, which either produce giant bubbles or streams of smaller ones. Some even produce square bubbles (with practice!). You can make a simple bubble machine by threading string through two plastic drinking straws and knotting it, to form a square with straws on two opposite sides and string on the others. Holding the straws, dip this gadget into a shallow tray of bubble mixture and then wave it gently through the air.

If you are using bubble blowers, make sure that everyone understands about blowing, rather than sucking. Experiment with lengths of plastic tubing and bowls of water and washing-up liquid — you will have time to see if people are sucking, and blowing will produce a satisfying number of bubbles on the surface of the water.

Dough

Dough, homemade with flour and water not the commercial playdough, is a wonderful medium — you can squidge it through your fingers, knead it, pummel it, cut it up, and then put it all back together again. When you are making a fresh batch of dough, don't make it somewhere else and then present it to the people who are going to use it — involve them in the making. They can feel the silky flour, stir in the water, knead the dough and then use it. Similarly, if you are going to colour the dough don't mix it in ready for use — make a depression in the dough, with your finger, add a few drops of food colouring, close the dough over it and let people knead it. The colour will gradually spread through the dough with a marble effect, until it is finally uniformly coloured.

There are various recipes for dough:

- 2 cups plain flour
- 1 cup salt
- 2 teaspoons cooking oil

- water to bind

Mix the dry ingredients together then add the oil and the water gradually. Knead until the dough is smooth. The salt is added to improve the keeping qualities of the dough and to discourage eating. However, it is not always a good idea — the high salt level may be uncomfortable for people with very dry skin and people may still eat the dough, despite the salt.

- 700 g self-raising flour
- 300 ml water

Mix the ingredients together and knead. This dough won't keep long, but it has a wonderful elastic texture and is very stretchy.

Experiment with other flours, e.g. wholemeal or strong plain flour, to create doughs with different properties.

- 1 mug plain flour
- $\frac{1}{2}$ mug salt
- 1 tablespoon cooking oil
- 1 tablespoon cream of tartar

Mix the dry ingredients together in a saucepan and then stir in the liquids. Cook over a low heat, stirring all the time, until the dough leaves the side of the pan (about 5 minutes). Remove from the heat and allow to cool slightly. Turn out onto a floured surface and knead until smooth. This dough will keep for several weeks.

When you have made your dough, you can add colour (using food colourings), smell (using mixed spice powder or food essences) and texture (knead dry lentils or rice into the dough).

This last receipe is not for a dough, as such, but it produces an incredible tactile material:

- 500 g cornflour
- 400 ml water

Place the cornflour in a large bowl and add sufficient water to produce a thick consistency. You now have an amazing substance which will behave partly as a liquid and partly as a solid. Hit the surface of the mixture with your fist and it is solid, rest your hand on the surface and it will sink into the liquid. Break off a piece and roll it into a ball on the palm of your hand — it will run away through your fingers. You can add food colouring and essences, if you wish, but most people find it quite fascinating as it is!

Paint

This section looks at activities using paint and includes some ideas for making pictures using materials other than paint (collage, etc.) In any art or craft activity it is essential to remember that the *process* is as important as the *end product*. The object is not to make things to please other people, but to please oneself. That said, it is important to value and display all work produced, not just the things we think are good.

We start with finger paint, which leads on from the messy activities described in the section above. It is possible to buy commercial finger paints but it is easy to make your own:

1. Mix equal amounts of plain flour and powder paint, add cold water until the mixture is thick and smooth.
2. Mix wallpaper paste (not one containing fungicide) to a thick consistency and add powder paint.
3. Mix powder paint with PVA glue (from educational catalogues).
4. Add texture to finger paints by mixing in sand, dry lentils or rice.
5. Add smells to different colours of paint, for extra sensory stimulation or for people with visual impairment, using food essences.
6. Use edible finger paints — tomato ketchup, mustard sauce, bread sauce, etc. or different flavours of Angel Delight, creamed rice, jam, fruit yogurts.

Finger painting can be done on Formica topped tables, plastic sheeting, or the glossy paper used for printing photographs (sometimes available from scrap banks — see chapter 10 — or direct from photographic developers and printers). Of course, it's not just for hands, feet can be used as well or various tools. Spread out the paint and make patterns using forks, combs, pieces of dowel and cardboard 'combs' (stiff cardboard strips with various cuts made along one edge).

When a pattern or a particular combination of colours has been created, a print can be taken by placing a piece of paper on top of the paint, gently pressing and peeling off the paper.

Ready mixed paints or powder paints (mixed with a little water and PVA glue, so that they are not too runny) can be used in various ways:

1. With brushes — toothbrushes, nailbrushes, shaving brushes, washing-up mops, scrubbing brushes, household paint brushes, sponges attached to pieces of dowel. Slip lengths of foam pipe lagging (from DIY stores) over the handles to make them easier to grasp.
2. With decorating rollers — various textures are available from DIY stores (they are used to produce different paint effects, or with Artex). Radiator rollers are smaller than ordinary rollers, and have a longer handle.
3. Bottle painting — suspend washing-up liquid bottles full of paint upside down above large sheets of paper, swing the bottle back and forth. Make a simple cradle (out of a wire coathanger) to hold the bottle, so that it is easier to swap bottles over to change colours.
4. Plastic deodorant bottles make excellent alternatives to large felt pens — prise off the roller ball, wash the bottle, fill with paint and replace the top.
5. Place different colours of dry powder paint in plastic pepper pots. Wet some paper and sprinkle on the powder paints, which will spread on the damp surface.

6. Spinning painting — use an old record player turntable (with all the electrical parts removed, so that it can be spun by hand), or a plastic 'Lazy Susan'. Place it in a large box, a plastic litter tray (from pet shops) or a Tidy Sheet (from Lakeland Plastics) to contain the paint, which will fly everywhere. Cut a circle of paper to fit the turntable, anchor it down with a piece of Blutac, and spray the paper with water. Set the turntable spinning and drip runny paint onto the paper to create very attractive patterns.

7. Marbling — special marbling inks are available but you can use powder paints mixed with cooking oil. Fill a plastic seed tray or litter tray with water, to a depth of about 3 cm. Float different colours of paint on the water. Gently float a piece of white paper on the surface of the water and remove it. Draw a thread, a feather or a fine skewer across the surface of the water to change the pattern of the paints.

8. Rolling paintings — place a piece of paper in the bottom of a biscuit tin, or a plastic seed or litter tray. Drop some paint on the paper then roll a marble or a small rubber ball across the surface of the paper (by tilting the tin or tray) to make a pattern.

9. Blowing paint — place runny paint on a piece of paper and create patterns by blowing through a straw, or using a hairdryer or the nozzle of a foot operated pump (from camping shops, for inflating airbeds).

10. Stencils — commercial ones, or homemade from thin plywood, hardboard or thick card. You can also use a wire baking tray, a plastic sink mat or stencils from cake decorating shops.

11. Spatter painting — dip an old toothbrush or nailbrush in paint and hold it over a piece of paper. Run a finger through the bristles. Paint will spatter on the paper (and everywhere else!).

12. 'Stained glass windows' — mix plenty of PVA glue with powder paint and use this to paint on thick polythene. Stick it to a window to see the 'stained glass' effect.

13. Leaves — paint the vein side of leaves and press them onto paper. When dry, the paper leaves can be cut out and used in collages.

14. Printing — use fairly thick paint for this. Place the paint in a large shallow tray, or soak a flat piece of foam sponge with the paint (like an ink pad). All kinds of objects can be used for printing:
    sponge shapes,
    lids from containers,
    cotton reels,
    wooden blocks with string glued on in various patterns,
    vegetables — cut a potato in half and carve various shapes in the surface. Try different vegetables such as a cabbage or a cauliflower floret cut in half.
    blocks of expanded polystyrene (packing material) — create random shapes in the surface by dropping nail varnish onto the polystyrene, to dissolve it.

Those are some of the things we can do with paint, but what do we paint on? A wide range of papers is available from the educational suppliers. When money is tight, it is tempting to use old computer paper and other scraps but it is important to give people experience with different types of paper — both the good quality and the cheaper alternatives. Offcuts of paper and card are often available from printers or scrap banks (see chapter 10).

Other interesting surfaces are corrugated cardboard, bubble plastic, fabrics and wallpaper (especially the embossed ones). Don't forget three-dimensional shapes as well — cardboard boxes and the tubes from carpets make an interesting change from flat pieces of paper.

PVA glue has been mentioned several times and it is worth reminding ourselves what a useful medium it is for art and craft work. Mixing powder paint with PVA glue and a little water produces a paint which will stick to smooth surfaces and has a shiny, hard wearing finish. PVA glue thinned with water can be used to glaze finished paintings or models made of plaster or self-hardening clay. It can also be added to papier mâché or plaster to increase strength. And, of course, PVA glue also sticks paper, card and fabrics.

Collage pictures can be created using various materials:

1. Sand patterns — try silver sand on black paper or tray, coloured sands on white paper or tray. Permanent pictures can be made by spreading PVA glue on paper and sprinkling the sand onto it. Coloured sand can be made by mixing sand with thin paint, allowing it to dry and sieving the sand.
2. Spread glue on pieces of card and sprinkle on various substances — glitter, rice, pearl barley, oats, crushed egg shells (paint the shells before crushing them), sequins, dried herbs, tea, paprika, chocolate vermicelli, 'hundreds and thousands'.
3. Make a picture by sticking different pulses and pasta shapes on a piece of black card.
4. Use PVA glue to stick cotton string in various patterns (wavy lines, coils, etc.) until the whole of the card is covered. The string can be left in its natural state, or dyed before use.
5. Make a three-dimensional collage using shallow boxes, tubes, plastic tubs.
6. Make a montage, using pictures cut or torn from magazines, or family photographs.
7. Make a collage of different types of paper, stuck down with wallpaper paste or PVA glue — patterned wrapping paper, textured wallpaper, tissue paper, sweet wrappers, silver foil, sandpaper, doilleys.
   Or use different fabrics — chiffon, coloured tights, lace, net, satin, velvet, tweed, fur fabric, leather, lurex, patterned cotton. The fabric can be pleated, crumpled or frayed and sequins, buttons or beads may be added.

Clay

Clay can be used in various ways, both for exploration and for creating objects. Ordinary clay is fired in a kiln and decorated by applying glazes, to produce durable items such as mugs. However, clay can also be left to dry and decorated with water-based paints and the resulting models will survive well. Self-hardening clay is more expensive but is easier to use and decorate. Many of the same activities can be done with a type of dough which is then baked:

- 4 cups flour
- 1-2 cups salt
- 1 cup water

Mix the dry ingredients together then add the water gradually, adding a little more if necessary to form a firm dough. Knead. Cut into shapes or make models. Place on a baking sheet and bake in a moderate oven (Mark 4/ 180° C) for about an hour, until lightly brown and firm. Remove from the oven and allow to cool (the shapes will harden further as they cool). The dough shapes can then be painted and varnished.

Various other modelling materials are available now (from craft shops and educational catalogues), some have interesting smells and colours, including fluorescent.

Clay, or the other modelling materials, can be rolled, bashed, squeezed, forced through a garlic press or potato ricer, or it can have objects pressed into it to create patterns. Models, whether abstract or representational, can be created. Jewellery can be made — roll round or cylindrical beads of clay and push them onto a knitting needle to make a hole through them. When dry, the beads can be painted and varnished.

An interesting group project is to make a decorative panel. Roll a slab of clay to an even thickness — place a piece of thin square-section wood on either side of the clay to act as guides for the rolling pin. Cut tiles from the clay, choosing shapes which will fit together — square, rectangle, hexagon, or triangle. Decorate the tiles by adding more clay to make raised designs, or by pressing objects into the tiles. When the clay has hardened, paint and varnish the tiles. Arrange them in a pattern and glue them to a piece of hardboard, using contact adhesive.

Puppets

There is something very special about puppets. Slip a glove puppet on your hand and it acquires a life and a character of its own. Watching it, we forget that it is being animated by the person on the other end of the arm! For most people, it is better to avoid stringed puppets as they are difficult to operate satisfactorily and their strings are easily tangled.

There are many excellent glove puppets available commercially:

1. Fluppets (toy shops) — realistic animal puppets, a good size for adult hands.
2. Sheep puppet (Dormouse Designs) — a large black and white sheep which makes a 'baaing' noise when you raise his head.

3. Multicultural puppets (Ann Johnson) — well-made puppets with authentic hairstyles and clothes.

Glove puppets are good fun if you can move your fingers to animate them, but they are frustrating if you cannot. Look for oven gloves in the form of animals (available from kitchen shops). An up and down movement of an arm can make the frog jump, a sideways movement makes the fish swim, and thus everyone can join in the activity.

You can also make your own puppets, and there are several books available which give instructions. Giant puppets can be made using a fabric-conditioner bottle as the head. Hold the bottle upside down, by the handle and mark a face on the side of the bottle. Add a hat and flowing robes with a broom handle as the arms, or a stuffed body with arms and legs.

See chapter 11 for details of suppliers and books.

7

Handling Objects

This chapter considers a whole range of objects to handle, from things to fiddle with through to equipment for more purposeful use — fitting together, turning, and so on.

Things to Fiddle With

Here are some simple ideas to start with:

1. Exploring bags: this idea uses the net bags which are intended to hold tights and delicate underwear in the washing machine. These bags are available from hardware stores or Lakeland Plastics. I have two bags — one contains balls of different sizes and weights (some soft, some hard, some which make a noise). The other bag contains various objects (a pan scourer, a soap holder with rubber suckers, a plastic rod and a ring from old toys, a cotton reel, and so on).

   These bags are an ideal way of presenting a range of items to be explored without any worries about whether items are too small and may be swallowed, because they are all safely held in the bag. If you think people may be able to undo the zip, you can sew some running stitches along the flap of netting which covers the zip.

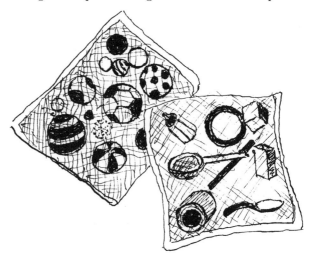

2. Strong cardboard tube, about 3 cm diameter (from a roll of plastic bags). Place two or three marbles in the tube. Cut two circles of thick card to cover the ends of the tube and secure them with plenty of PVC tape. Cover the tube with self-adhesive diffraction foil (for visual stimulation) or Vivelle (for tactile stimulation). Tilting the tube produces a noise plus the feeling of weight being transferred from one end of the tube to the other.

3. Take a length of large-diameter plastic tubing. Drill holes through it at intervals. Thread pieces of coloured, plastic-covered clothes-line and strong elastic through the holes, with coloured plastic beads and bells threaded on them. Knot the ends of the line or elastic and put a dab of Araldite glue on each knot.

4. Plastic bowl of balls (see chapter 8 for a range of balls) to stir around, grasp and pass from hand to hand.

5. Plastic bowl of household objects — sieve, funnel, pastry cutters, brushes, etc. — to handle, fit together, and so on.

6. The mother of a young autistic man told me that the best present she ever gave him was a container full of plastic clothes pegs. He could rummage through them, sort the different colours, clip them round the top of the container or onto a piece of cardboard or a length of plastic-covered clothes-line.

7. Basket of wooden objects to handle. Different woods have different textures, grains, colours and even smells. My collection includes an egg cup, napkin ring, pastry brush, lemon reamer, carved animals (dolphin and frog), smooth 'eggs', irregular shapes, a wooden apple (from Lakeland Plastics or craft shops) with apple oil to scent it, a wooden spoon and a small box with a pierced lid (for pot pourri). This collection is ideal for restless hands.

8. Interest boxes: themed collections of objects provide good rummaging material, but also objects which can be explored, sorted and discussed. Themes could include sea shells (both natural ones collected from the beach and polished ones), metal objects (bunches of keys, metal puzzles, etc.), scraps of fabrics with interesting textures, brushes (pastry, hair, tooth, nail, paint, scrubbing and make-up brushes), realistic silk and plastic flowers, kitchen gadgets (pastry wheel, hand-operated whisk, timer, etc.), animals (I find that the domestic and wild animals made by Playmobil, from educational catalogues, are the most realistic) and transport (model cars, buses, lorries, planes, boats).

9. Large coat buttons threaded on a loop of strong, round elastic.

10. Thick elastic bands stretched over an empty cardboard box. Make a nice 'twang' and thumping noise if you can pick them up with your finger. Stretching the bands across an old picture frame makes them easier to pluck, but you don't get the same noise.

11. Salad spinner: place cat balls (hard plastic balls with bells inside), plastic cotton reels and a bunch of bells (tied loosely to the inside of the inner cage, so that they cannot be swallowed if the lid is removed) in the spinner and replace the lid. If you turn the handle (you need to be fairly strong to get it going), you will get noise plus a rumbling vibration.

12. 'Bran tub' games: play hide-and-seek games by hiding objects in a variety of 'tubs' and encouraging people to rummage for them. The objects can be hidden under polystyrene packing shapes (don't use if there is any danger of them being eaten), crumpled paper, leaves, sand, foil coffee bags, lentils, strips of survival blanket, or water with bubbles on it (use objects which sink).

13. Activity boards: commercial versions are available but there are many DIY ideas you can try:
    - Stuff socks with various textures (polystyrene packing shapes, pieces of survival blanket, bubble plastic, cellophane, etc.), thread them through the smallest possible hole in a wooden board and knot firmly at the back.
    - Do the same with the legs of coloured tights: place some filling in the toe, pass it through a hole and knot at the back. Thread it back through a hole, put in a different filling, thread through and knot. Repeat until the leg is used up, ending with a large knot on the back. Leave the 'sausages' filled with textures fairly loose so that fingers can explore them easily.
    - Thread various objects on strong, thick elastic and knot the elastic at the back of the board, pulling it tight so that the objects stand upright like stalks, and stapling the elastic to the underside of the board, using a staple gun. Objects can include beads, cotton reels, plastic tubing, plastic film canisters (drill through base and lid, place bell inside, glue lid on), various shapes of caps from bottles, wooden rings (from craft or pet shops), plastic pan scrubbers, practice golf balls and Gamester balls.
    - Glue a large wooden bead on the end of a piece of thick nylon rope, using Araldite. Thread the rope through the board and up through another hole, glue a bead on the other end. Make the holes large enough for the rope to move easily and use sufficient rope so that the beads can be pulled backwards and forwards. Make several of these pairs of beads and match the colours, so that when the green bead is pulled the other green bead hits the board, and so on.

DIY Ideas

Here are some more detailed instructions for making equipment:

Feely Tabard (Roma Lear)

In 'Play Helps' Roma shows how to make aprons or tabards to which various objects can be attached. These are ideal for people who have difficulty handling objects, because there is always something for your hands to find, if an item is dropped it won't fall out of reach, and nobody else can take it away.

Tabards are better than aprons because there are no tapes to get tangled and it is easier to remove a tabard quickly if necessary.

Choose a rectangular piece of fabric in an interesting texture (avoid bold patterns as the objects will not show up) approximately 40 cm wide and 1 m long. Fold over one third of the fabric and cut a hole to fit over the head. Hem the sides and ends of the fabric and bind the neck with tape.

The shorter end of the fabric is the back of the tabard — if you spend long periods of time sitting in a chair, it can be uncomfortable to have fabric rucked up and sticking in your back.

Make two pockets at the bottom of the front. These can hold small objects to be explored and favourite treasures, such as a sweetpaper or shoelace, which may get swept up and thrown away if dropped on the floor.

Machine a piece of tape or carpet braid across the wrong side of the front, about one third of the way down. On the right side, machine three tape loops, sewing through the reinforcing tape on the back. Attach objects to the tape loops (hair roller, bell cage, spoons, rings, etc.) using short lengths of cord or tape. Remember to change the objects frequently, preferably introducing one new object at a time, to be discovered among the familiar ones.

Roller Doodle Loop (Roma Lear)

Roma describes this idea in 'More Play Helps' and, once again, I think this is an excellent item for adults as well as children.

A series of loops of material (like miniature roller towels) are made to slide over a wheelchair tray so that there is something to explore and handle, at times when individual attention is not possible.

Cut strips of fabric approximately 30 cm wide and long enough to make a tube which will be a loose fit on the tray. Machine the ends together and hem the edges. Choose a range of plain colours for the loops, so that they will provide a good background for the textures and objects you are going to attach.

Look for good visual contrast and a variety of interesting textures or sounds:

- Patchwork of textures
- Bath plug chain (oversew between each 'ball', using strong button thread)
- Upholstery fringing
- Appliqued flowers (cut from floral fabrics and machined on with zig-zag stitches)
- Interesting shaped and metallic buttons, bells (securely sewn on, with a piece of reinforcing fabric behind the material and using strong button thread)
- A circle of fabric, zig-zagged to the material and enclosing a flat plastic squeaker (from craft shops)

89

Remember that everything must be very firmly attached and safe, because these doodle loops are intended for unsupervised use.

Feely Fish (JD, inspired by Roma Lear)

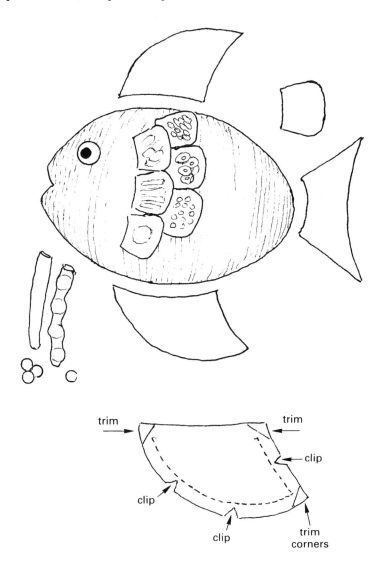

trim   trim

clip

clip

clip   trim
              corners

There is a design in 'Play Helps' for a feely tortoise and Roma mentions that you could use the same idea for a fish.

To my mind, a tortoise looks like a child's soft toy so I set out to make a fish which would look like a designer cushion or soft sculpture but which would still offer all the 'feelies'. The very first time I exhibited the fish, someone commented that she would happily use it with adults — which pleased me, as you can imagine!

I chose a thin cotton fabric for the scales, fins etc. and a fine needlecord in a toning colour for the body of the fish. It is important to choose attractive colours; avoid using scraps of different fabrics — many people associate patchwork effects with children's equipment, for some reason.

Draw a flat fish (like plaice) shape on thin paper and use this to cut out the two body pieces; cut a 'V' shape for the mouth.

Work out how many scales you can fit on your fish; cut pairs of scale shapes, an upper and lower fin, and a tail from the thin cotton (see diagram). Match pairs of scales, right sides together, and machine round the curved edge of each pair. Turn right side out and place a different 'feelie' in each scale (e.g. rice, dried peas, pasta shapes, washers, coins, Rawlplugs, buttons, a flat plastic squeaker — from craft shops). Turn under the raw edges and pin across the straight edge of each scale.

Position the scales on the right side of one of the body pieces, slightly overlapping them, and making sure that they are all within the 1 cm seam allowance which you will take when you machine the body. When you are satisfied with the arrangement, attach the scales to the body by machining across each one, near to the straight edge.

Decide where the eye will go and sew it on. The most effective fish eye is a small black button sewn on top of a slightly larger pearly white one. If you are worried about buttons, use circles of felt.

Machine round the curved edges of each fin and the tail, with right sides together. Clip the curved seam allowance at intervals and trim the points. Turn right side out. Place several layers of bubble plastic in each fin and the tail. Make sure that the plastic extends beyond the raw edges of the material, so that you will machine through the plastic when you attach the fins and tail (this helps them to stand out stiffly from the fish, rather than flopping).

Make two tubes from the thin material and place three or four marbles in each tube. You will have to use trial and error to make the tubes — the size will depend on the size of your marbles. Your aim is to achieve a tube which will hold the marbles in a single line but which will allow them to slide up and down easily. These tubes represent the 'dangly bits' (I don't know what they are called!) which you see under the mouths of some tropical fish; moving the marbles backwards and forwards is similar to fiddling with worry beads.

Now assemble the fish: tack the two body pieces together with right sides facing each other and with the fins, tail and tubes sandwiched between them (open edges lined up with the edges of the body pieces, so that they will be in the correct positions when you turn the fish right side out. Make sure that none of the scales will be caught in the seam. Machine around the fish, with a 1 cm seam allowance, leaving a 10 cm gap which will enable you to turn the fish the right way out.

Turn the fish right side out. Stuff with polyester stuffing, working some stuffing into the points of the mouth area using the end of a pencil. Stuff the fish fairly firmly, but maintain the flatness of it. Close the gap with hand stitches.

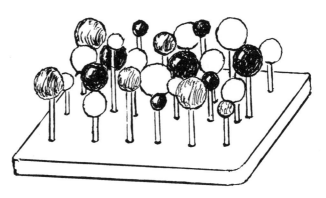

Wobbleboard (JD)

I designed this piece of equipment, when I was running a toy library, for someone who was just beginning to reach out and touch things. I wanted her to get an immediate response of movement and noise, plus a tactile sensation. Although designed for someone with very profound disabilities, the Wobbleboard has been popular with a wide range of people — indeed it seems to have similar properties to worry beads!

The Wobbleboard consists of a heavy wooden base with wooden balls on lengths of springy wire, which move at the slightest touch.

The materials you will need are

- A piece of plywood, approximately 3 cm thick. The size and the shape are up to you — you could choose a square, rectangle, circle, or an irregular wavy shape.
- Wooden balls: these are sold (in various sizes — 2 cm and 3 cm diameter are best for this project) by some timber yards or are available by mail order from D. & J. Simons and Sons Ltd. (122/150 Hackney Road, London E2 7QL; Tel 071-739 3744). You could use wooden threading beads instead (not plastic — the glue won't stick properly).
- Curtain wire (plastic coated, sold for net curtains)
- Paint and varnish
- Drill (electric or hand), drill bit, countersink drill
- G cramp
- Sandpaper or orbital sander

Method

Mark the positions for the holes (for the wire) on the plywood. Don't go mad — about 30 wooden balls will be plenty for most purposes. Position the holes so that the balls will not be touching when stationary, but will hit each other when they are moving.

Choose a drill size which is right for your curtain wire — the wire should fit into the hole easily, but not loosely, so that there is room for some glue round the wire. Drill the holes. Don't go all the way through, only about two thirds of the way. If you are worried about going too far, wrap a piece of masking tape round the drill to indicate the depth you should reach. Open out each hole using the countersink drill (this will enable you to get a good pool of glue round each wire). Sand the board until it is completely smooth, rounding the edges and any corners. Brush off any loose sawdust and apply several coats of silk finish varnish.

Now drill a hole half way through each wooden ball, using the same sized drill and the countersink. You will need someone to help you with this stage, one person to hold the balls (in the G cramp) and one to do the drilling. This must be done with great care — use a hand drill unless you are very skilled with an electric drill. Hold each ball in the G cramp. Place a crumpled scrap of kitchen paper on either side of the ball to reduce the damage done by the cramp as you tighten it up. If you are using a Workmate, rest the ball on one of the holes in the top, for more support.

Hold the drill vertically, so that the hole goes to the centre of the ball. If you are using an electric drill, start with a slow speed until the drill bit bites on the curved surface. Access to a drill stand (which holds the drill vertically) would be very useful.

If you are using wooden beads instead of balls, you will avoid this difficult piece of drilling — simply place some Araldite in one end of each bead (using a scrap piece of curtain wire to push it in) and leave it to harden completely.

Now make the 'lollipops': cut lengths of curtain wire; vary the lengths — short, stubby wires will move differently from longer ones — but don't make them too long, or the balls will droop. Trim a small piece of plastic off each end of each wire, using a craft knife, so that the glue will come into contact with the wire as well as the plastic. Mix some Araldite according to the instructions, scoop up some glue on the end of the wire, insert it in the ball or bead and twist it round gently to produce a smooth 'collar' of glue. If you are using Araldite Rapid, only mix a small quantity at a time, as it will harden very quickly. Attach the rest of the balls or beads to the wires in the same way.

If you are using beads they will already be coloured, so you don't need to paint them, but you may wish to give them a couple of coats of varnish for extra protection. If you are using balls, paint them (see chapter 2 for information on paints you can use) and then varnish. The wire attached to each ball makes it easy to hold for painting and varnishing and you can poke the wires into a block of polystyrene or florist's foam to keep the 'lollipops' upright while they dry.

Now place the 'lollipops' in the holes in the board and move them around until you are happy with the arrangement of colour and heights. Glue each wire in place as before.

Finally, a word about the strength of this piece of equipment. If you mix Araldite correctly, it is one of the strongest glues available. The Wobbleboard is suitable for use by anyone who is not strong enough to grasp a wooden ball and pull it so hard that the curtain wire starts to unravel. In normal use, a piece of curtain wire may start to break off just above the glue in the board — because of metal fatigue. If this happens, cut the wire off, smooth any roughness with a file, and cover the spot with a smooth blob of Araldite. Go on using your Wobbleboard with one less ball.

Here are a few simple ideas for more skilful handling activities:

1. Drawer Organizer (Lakeland Plastics): this consists of plastic strips which slot together to make compartments in a drawer or shallow plastic tray. Use for sorting activities.
2. Use a cutlery tray for sorting activities.
3. Use a desk tidy (a cluster of plastic tubes, for storing pens, etc.) for fitting activities, placing lengths of dowel or pencils in the various tubes.
4. Use a pencil holder (shaped like a hedgehog, with plastic spikes) — fit pencils between the spikes.
5. Stack wooden napkin rings, small decorating rollers or large hair rollers on a paper towel holder (a vertical wooden pole on a stand).
6. Make a threading board: drill holes, about 3 cm in diameter, in a piece of thin plywood using a flat wood bit and an electric drill. Thread lengths of clear plastic tubing or garden hose (soft plastic, not the stiff, ridged type) through the holes.
7. Finer threading: buy a square of pegboard (hardboard with small holes drilled all over it). Thread sparkly or fluorescent shoelaces through the holes to make patterns. You can make a stand to hold the pegboard, so that both hands can be used for threading. Position two lengths of square section softwood on a piece of plywood, parallel to each other, with a gap between them into which the pegboard will slot. Attach the wood to the plywood using wood glue and panel pins.
8. 'Sewing cards': draw various shapes or pictures on the smooth side of hardboard squares. Drill holes at intervals round the outlines of the shapes. Paint the shapes. Use earth-wire sleeving (hollow plastic tubing, sold in DIY stores and electrical suppliers) to thread round the outlines. These boards can be used in the stand described above.
9. Ask local shops to save the plastic tubes from the centre of till rolls. Sometimes they are different colours. If not, paint them with enamel paint or stick textures on them (using UHU or Bostik). Use them as threading beads, with lengths of plastic covered clothes line.
10. Collect old bead seats (for car seats). Cut the threads to release the wooden beads and use them for threading. Make your own bead curtains for doorways by threading the beads on strong fishing line or cord.

Commercial Equipment

There is a very wide range of equipment available , both in the educational catalogues and from the specialist suppliers. I have used this section to highlight particular items which I think are useful.

1. Sensory Bead Curtain (TFH): lengths of bath-plug chain, a wonderful heavy, almost silky sensation when you run your hand through the curtain.

2. Roller Run (TFH): small wooden item. Marbles run down the slopes and bounce on some xylophone keys at the bottom to produce a musical ending.

3. Musical Fantasy (Kouvalias, from Raven): music box which rotates as it plays, plus balls on springs to fiddle with.

4. Magical Daisies (Kouvalias, from Raven): wooden flowerheads on springs bounce and a bell rings, as the wheeled platform moves along.

5. Chimeabout (Edu-play): all the Edu-play items are excellent, the ones described here are some of my favourites. The Chimeabout has beautiful stained wooden chimes and bells on a stand. The slightest touch produces movement and sound.

6. Mirror Chimeabout (Edu-play): Strips of mirror Perspex, backed with blue and red Perspex, plus bells on a stand. Both Chimeabouts are also available as hanging mobiles.

7. Clacking Windmill (Edu-play): a double windmill, very easy to spin. This is one of the few items I can think of which actually gets more interesting as it slows down — the wooden pieces on the arms of the windmills make the most clacking noise then.

8. Mirror Marble Wheel (Edu-play): a ship's wheel with mirror behind Perspex. Nylon cups and marbles between the two layers move as the wheel is spun.

9. Diffraction Tube Roller/Shaker (Edu-play): an adult-sized and appropriate rattle incorporating diffraction foil.

10. Diffraction Tube Ladder (Edu-play): different colours of foil in tubes. The ladder can be used at two different angles.

11. Helter Skelter Loopie (Mike Ayres & Co.): plastic balls posted in the top race down a clear plastic tube and appear in the tray at the bottom. Good for group use.

12. Floor Cogboard/Wall Cogboard (Mike Ayres & Co.): large wooden cogs can be positioned on various pegs. Turning one cog will make all the others which are interlocking turn as well.

13. One Armed Bandit Posting Box (TFH): large wooden posting box. Shapes reappear when the handle at the side is pulled. Beware! Objects other than balls can be posted into the box but will not come out when the handle is pulled. It's a fiddly job to get them out.

14. Sticklebricks (toy shops, educational catalogues): plastic bricks which fit together with their 'prickles'. Interesting texture, but they can be painful for people with sore or cracked skin on their hands.

15. Popoids (toy shops, educational catalogues): plastic concertina tubes which stretch with a popping noise. Discard the childish animal heads and use the tubes to fit into the other plastic shapes, or on their own for stretching and squashing.

16. Magnetic Blocks (educational catalogues): plastic blocks with metal surfaces and magnets. Very low effort construction material.

17. Velcro Building Set and Velcro Activity Board (TFH): various shapes fit together and to the board by means of Velcro — always popular!

18. Magnadoodle (toy shops): works on the same principle as Etch a Sketch, but much easier to use and more spectacular results. Use the magnetic

pen to draw lines, spirals, loops, and the two magnetic shapes to make bold patterns.

Inset Boards and Jigsaws

Most educational and specialist catalogues include some inset boards and jigsaws which are suitable for adults (see below) but there are several items which we can make ourselves.

Texture Inset Board (JD)

There are very few commercial texture-matching boards and those that exist never give you a large enough piece of texture to explore! Also, the textures are permanently fixed to the wood or plastic but they will quickly become dirty, so you don't want anything too permanent.

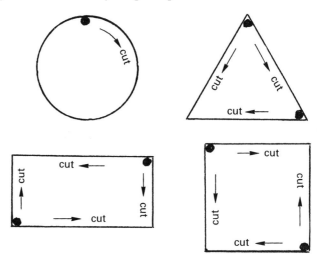

Choose two pieces of plywood which are the same size. Cut circles (or squares, or different shapes) out of one piece of wood. To do this, drill a hole in the edge of the circle which is just large enough for the blade of the electric jigsaw to pass through. Cut round the circle. If you are cutting out a triangle, you will need a hole in two of the points, in order to cut it out. If the shape is a square or a rectangle, you will need a hole in two opposite corners.

Whenever you are cutting out geometric shapes for an inset board, cut them as accurately as possible and sand them if necessary, so that they will fit easily — a circle should fit in any orientation, an equilateral triangle in three orientations, a square in four, and a rectangle or oval in two. If a shape will only fit in one way, it will be very frustrating for the user.

When you have cut out your shapes, mark their positions on the base board. Choose your textures and cut pieces to fit under each hole, plus 2 cm allowance all round. Position the textures and anchor them down by applying a little Copydex around the edges only. Screw the base board to the top board, so that the textures are held firmly in place.

Attach a small wooden doorknob (from DIY stores) to each inset shape and stick on the appropriate texture, using Copydex.

When the textures on the board are dirty, remove the screws, separate the boards and replace the textures with new pieces.

Inset Board

This was made by a member of staff at the RNIB's Condover Hall School, when she was studying on the in-service training course.

Make a wooden inset board with four different large shapes — circle, square, rectangle and triangle — as described above. Use four different plain colours of cotton or polycotton fabric for the board, not different textures. Cut the four shapes — cylinder, square, rectangle and a piece with a triangular cross-section — from foam plastic, using a serrated bread knife. Sew a cover for each shape, using the appropriate coloured fabric.

Simple Jigsaws (JD)

1. Buy a solid wooden breadboard (circular, with a groove or similar decoration round the edge). Using an electric jigsaw, cut the board into five pieces by cutting wavy lines across the board. Start and finish each cut with the blade approximately at right angles to the edge of the board, so that none of the pieces have sharp points. Sand the cut edges and apply three or four coats of silk varnish for a hard–wearing finish. You now have a push-together jigsaw and you can identify the right side of each piece by the edge decoration or groove.

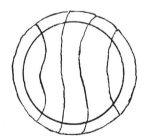 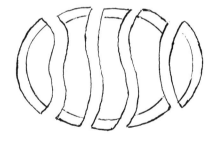

2. Buy a solid, wooden, rectangular chopping board. Cut it into six pieces with wavy edges, as on page 98. This jigsaw will need something to indicate which is the right side of the pieces, otherwise it will be very difficult indeed! You could paint a pattern or picture onto the wood, and then varnish it. Or you could use self-adhesive Vivelle, diffraction foil or glitter paper (all available from Rompa) to make a pattern.

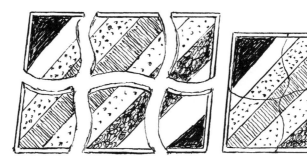

Interlocking Jigsaws (JD)

You won't be able to make small-piece interlocking jigsaws unless you can use a coping saw (a handsaw which can turn round tight corners) or you have access to a model maker's bandsaw (which has a very fine blade). However, for many people a large-piece jigsaw will be more appropriate and these can be made using an electric jigsaw.

Posters of pop stars, racing cars, etc. can be used, or photographs which are relevant to the person who will use the jigsaw — themselves, family, pets, their home or a group of friends, for example. Choose a photograph which is sharply focused, so that it will enlarge well. Some developers offer poster-sized prints at reasonable cost, otherwise enlargement by colour photocopying is not too expensive.

Stick the picture to a piece of plywood, using PVA glue spread evenly to ensure that all parts of the picture are stuck down. Allow the glue to dry completely. Cover the whole picture with tracing or greaseproof paper (sticking strips together with masking tape to make a wide enough piece, if necessary). Wrap the paper over the edges of the plywood and stick it to the underside with masking tape. Draw your jigsaw pieces on the paper, in pencil, making sure that all the curves of the knuckle joints are open and gradual (if they are too tight the saw blade won't be able to get round them). Look at a commercial wooden jigsaw, if necessary, to work out how the pieces should fit together.

Use the finest blade in your electric jigsaw and start cutting out the pieces. Keep the base plate of the saw flat on the wood at all times, so that the saw is cutting vertically — if you don't, the pieces won't fit together properly. The greaseproof paper will protect your picture from being scuffed by the base plate. Using an electric jigsaw is a bit like ironing — the iron is hot, but you decide when to move it. Similarly, the saw blade can be moving up and down quite quickly, but you decide how fast to push the saw forward. If you keep the saw blade moving at a reasonable speed, but only move the saw forward slowly, you will be surprised at the way it will go round the knuckle joints by gradually nibbling at the wood. If you move the saw too fast, you won't be able to follow your lines and you will probably break the blade.

Cutting the pieces will be much easier if you have a Workmate. You can position the wood so that you are cutting in the gap between the two halves of the top of the Workmate. Your wood will be supported on both sides, you can clamp it down using a G cramp (place a piece of scrap wood between your wood and the cramp, to avoid damaging your picture), and you can re-position your wood as necessary.

When you have cut all the pieces, sand the cut edges lightly and check that the picture is still firmly stuck to the wood. Apply a very thin coat of varnish all over the picture (don't let the paper get too wet) and the edges of the wood. Allow it to dry completely. Apply three more thin coats of varnish in the same way.

Commercial Jigsaws

The educational catalogues have ranges of wooden jigsaws with photographs of vehicles, people working, family celebrations and everyday situations. Many of these pictures show people from different races and cultures, but very few show people with disabilities taking part in ordinary life.

Beautiful stained wooden puzzles are available from some craft shops and fairs, many of the pictures are suitable. TFH and Rompa also supply some appropriate jigsaws.

Various inset boards are available from the catalogues, but they often have tiny plastic knobs which are useless. Pull these knobs off, using pliers, and replace them with:

- Plastic covered cup hooks
- Wooden door knobs
- Plastic golf tees ('professional' ones are the best shape) — drill a hole through the wooden shape which is large enough for the tee to fit through. Open out the hole (on the wrong side) with a countersink drill. Push the tee through and melt the plastic against a hot iron or a soldering iron, so that it forms a 'plug' in the countersunk hole.
- A steel drawing pin hammered into each shape until the head is flat against the wood. Stick a small round industrial magnet (from hardware stores) to a short length of broom handle or dowel, using contact adhesive, and use this to lift out the pieces.

Anchoring Things Down

Often, when we give people objects to handle and explore it is difficult to ensure that the object stays in the right place for them. It is very frustrating if you knock the object over, or it falls on the floor, as soon as you touch it and it doesn't exactly encourage exploration. There are various ways of anchoring things down:

1. Dycem — a roll is more convenient than the shaped mats, as you can cut exactly the piece you want.
2. 'Stay put' discs (from rehab catalogues) are usually used to hold dishes steady, but can be used for other objects as well.

3. Blutac or 'Sticky fixers' can be used as a temporary solution.
4. Soap holders (from hardware stores), with suckers, can be used to form a strong grip between two smooth, non-porous surfaces.
5. Velcro ('hook' pieces) can be stuck on the bottom of various items of leisure equipment and the table or tray covered with Expoloop (available from suppliers of display stands) or another suitable fabric to which the Velcro will stick. You could also use the Velcro Activity Board from TFH.
6. Magnetic tape can be attached to the bottom of objects which are then used on a metal surface (a suitable tray, baking sheet, or a commercial magnetic board).
7. Some wooden leisure items can be screwed to a larger piece of plywood, which can then be clamped to the table.
8. The Active Worksheets (see chapter 10) contain a design for an adjustable base, which will hold various objects, and a table clamp which holds trays for puzzles and mosaics.
9. A bicycle tyre on a table provides an area in which to work and prevents objects moving out of reach.
10. Rifton supply a Horizontal Suction Cup Handgrip, a piece of wood 30 cm long with a very strong suction cup at each end. This will attach firmly to any smooth, non-porous surface (vertical or horizontal) and a variety of objects can be tied to it. Keep the string or cord for each item fairly short so that the player does not become tangled in it.
11. Objects which will roll, or move by battery power, can be restricted by placing them in a large plastic litter tray (from pet shops) so that they remain in view and within reach. Conversely, battery powered items which find it hard to move on some types of carpet will move more freely in the tray.

Making Things Happen

One of our most important aims should be to enable people to make choices and to control their environment. In the context of leisure, this can be encouraged by linking a switch which the person can operate to a piece of equipment which she would like to be able to operate.

A range of excellent switches is available from QED, including a light pressure switch, a sturdier one, blow/suck switches and a tilt switch. They also supply battery adaptors, consisting of a metal disc (which slips into the battery compartment) connected to a socket into which the jack plug of the switch is inserted.

One advantage of the QED switches is that they are all fitted with large jack plugs (which are sturdier than the miniature ones); also, the same switches can be used to control a computer, so the user can progress from a simple battery powered object to accessing appropriate computer software.

Switches are available from other suppliers; for instance, TFH have a range of sturdy wooden switches but they are very bulky and many are fitted with miniature jack plugs, which are vulnerable to damage. There is an

Active Worksheet (see chapter 10) for a sliding switch, which is ideal for people who have difficulty controlling their jerky movements.

A switch can be used to control a battery-powered animal, such as Pudgey the Piglet (who walks, grunts and moves its tail), and this is a fun way of teaching the 'cause and effect' nature of a switch i.e. when I press the switch the pig moves; when I stop, it stops. A range of animals is available from Raven and TFH; they are also available in many toy shops.

Other animals are not controlled by an external switch. The Vibrating Spider (Raven, TFH) is a wonderfully hairy, black and yellow spider which moves sideways in response to sound (vocal or clapping hands). For those who cannot stand spiders, there is a red Vibrating Crab (Raven, Rompa) which behaves in the same way. Even more popular is the Runaway Hedgehog (Raven), which has a heat sensor in its back — as you go to stroke it, the hedgehog moves away.

Battery adaptors and switches may be used with a wide range of battery powered equipment, apart from animals. Small fans, a motorist's lamp (often with flashing orange lights), a siren (from bicycle shops) or a cassette recorder, for instance. If the person wants to listen to a cassette, a latching switch will be useful. This is a pressure switch which is pressed once for 'on' and again for 'off' — so the person doesn't have to press the switch all the time to listen to the music.

You may find that the wire of the battery adaptor stops the flap of the battery compartment closing properly. If so, melt a little 'nick' in the edge of the flap, using a soldering iron, so that the wire can pass through.

The most important point about using switches is that the person should have the switch she can operate, connected to the equipment she wants to control, and that she can decide when she wants to switch it on and off.

8

Games

This chapter looks at various types of games, some of which require equipment and some organization and others which are 'spur of the moment' activities. Some games are explicitly, or by implication, competitive but others are co-operative and can be enjoyed for the playing, rather than for the winning. Games are a good way of encouraging a group to work together and can help people to develop relationships and practise their social skills. However, the opposite effect will be achieved if the game is not chosen with care, taking into account the abilities and interests of the people involved.

DIY Ideas

Colour Matching Game (Roma Lear)

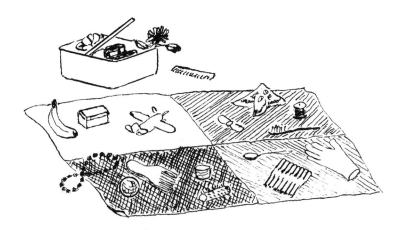

Roma describes making this game originally to teach the more unusual colours like pink, purple and brown. It consists of a mat made up of the colours chosen for the game and a collection of objects in the same colours. These can be placed on the correct sections of the mat, either as a solo activity or as a group game. I think it is an excellent game but I usually make it with the basic colours — red, blue, yellow and green — for first colour matching skills. It is a good piece of equipment because:

1. You can choose objects which are appropriate for the individual or group: sturdy or fragile, toys or everyday objects, familiar objects or not, and so on.
2. Handling and talking about the items and how they are used encourages group involvement and learning new words, signs or gestures.
3. It is a useful way of teaching that different shades of a colour are all called the same name — commercial colour matching games always use the same shade.
4. If a few pieces are lost, you can easily collect some more.

My mat is made of four knitted rectangles sewn together, but you could use plain fabrics instead. The collection of objects includes artificial flowers, toothbrush, comb, clothes-peg, card of buttons, string of beads, reel of sewing thread, coloured pencil, gift bow, bangle, Dinky car, plastic aeroplane, hair roller, nailbrush shaped like a frog and a strip of Rawlplugs (What are they? Do they make a noise if we blow them?).

Noughts and Crosses (JD)

I first made this game for my toy library, many years ago, and it proved popular both with people who wanted to play noughts and crosses and with those who just liked the noise of the Velcro ripping apart!

When I first made it, I used the same sized piece of Velcro on the board as on the noughts and crosses. Then I realized that you had to place the shapes very accurately to locate the Velcro, so now I have a larger patch on the board to make things easier.

Materials

- Board: cotton or polycotton, in a plain colour; polyester wadding
- Noughts: spotted fabric
- Crosses: gingham (checked) fabric
- 3 cm wide Velcro
- Ric-rac braid

Method

To make the board, cut two pieces of fabric 48 cm square. Place the right sides together and pin to a piece of wadding the same size. Machine round all four sides, with a 1.5 cm seam allowance, leaving a gap of 10 cm at the end of the fourth side. Trim the corners and turn right side out, through the gap you have left. Smooth the board flat and close the gap with hand stitching. The board should be 45 cm square. Pin pieces of the ric-rac braid in position to mark out nine 15 cm squares, turning under the ends of each piece to stop them fraying. Machine the braid to the board.

103

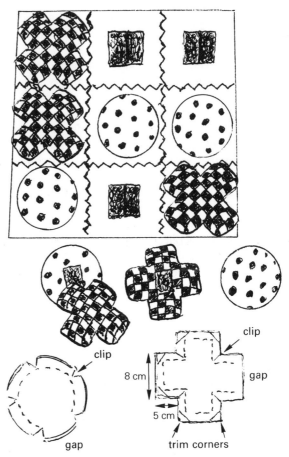

Cut 6 cm lengths of Velcro 'hooks' and position two pieces side by side in the middle of each playing square, to form a 6 cm square of Velcro. Machine in place.

Cut five pairs of circles, about 15 cm diameter (draw round a saucer), from the spotted fabric. Cut five pairs of crosses (see diagram for dimensions) from the gingham fabric. Machine a 3 cm piece of Velcro 'loops' in the centre of the right side of five circle and five cross pieces of fabric.

Pair up the circles, right sides together, and machine round them with a 1 cm seam allowance leaving a 4 cm gap. Clip the curve at intervals then turn them right side out, through the gap. Stuff with polyester stuffing and close the gaps with hand stitching.

Pair up the crosses and machine together in the same way, leaving the end of the last cross piece open. Trim the outer corners and clip the inner corners, turn right side out, stuff and sew up the gaps.

Large Draughts Board (JD)

This board uses coffee jar lids as the draughts and a board knitted in dark brown and beige squares. I wanted the board to look as much like an

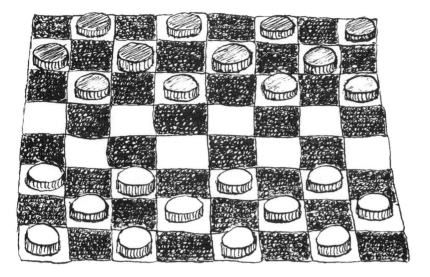

ordinary draughts board as possible, but you could use brighter colours for greater contrast if you want to. The board is worked in stocking stitch but you could work in a different stitch for each colour.

The number of stitches and rows you will need to form each square will depend on the thickness of your wool and what size needles you are using. Experiment to find the right size — I found that 20 stitches and 25 rows gave me a square on which the coffee jar lid fitted easily.

I find it easier to work the board in strips and then sew them together. Make the first square, then change to the other colour and continue alternating until you have completed eight squares. Cast off. Make seven more strips in the same way, remembering to start four strips with one colour and four with the other. Sew all the strips together.

Collect twelve coffee jar lids in each of two colours (e.g. brown and green) for the set of draughts and you're ready to play.

Non-competitive Race Game (Irma Mullins)

Irma, who is manager of Playtrac (see chapter 10), designed this game as a more adult version of the Snail's Race Game by Ravensburger. With most racetrack games, each player is hoping that her piece will reach the winning line first. In this game the players work together, taking it in turns to move whichever playing piece is indicated by the die.

You will need:

- a rectangular piece of plywood
- felt pens or paints to mark the racetrack
- six playing pieces — these could be six different model animals, or six vehicles (e.g. car, lorry, bus, ambulance, etc.)
- a 5 cm cube of wood (from an old set of building blocks)

Mark the six lanes of the racetrack on the plywood. I find it is better to keep the lanes separate (rather than adjacent to each other) so that everyone can see which lane is which. Make sure that each space is big enough for the animal or vehicle to stand on. Varnish the wood.

Make simple line drawings of each animal or vehicle, trying to make them look as like the object as possible. If you feel that you cannot draw them, find suitable pictures to trace. If the drawings are not the right size, reduce them on a photocopier until they will fit on the faces of the wooden cube. Stick the drawings on the cube, using PVA glue. Cover the cube with self-adhesive clear plastic, to protect the pictures.

Place the animals (or vehicles) on their starting spaces. Each player takes it in turn to throw the die and move whichever playing piece is indicated.

Performance Game (Lisa Corrick and Fiona Morrison)

This game was designed by Lisa and Fiona, when they were students on the BA (Hons) Professional Studies: Learning Difficulties course at Stockport College of Technology. I like it because it involves lots of action which can be enjoyed by players and spectators, and because the game can be adapted to suit the abilities and interests of the players.

The game consists of a large white sheet, on which the playing board is marked using laundry markers and fabric paints (see diagram). Machine pieces of Velcro 'hooks' round the edge of the sheet, on the underside, so that it will stick to the carpet and stop the sheet moving. Various props are placed in the centre of the board (these are described in more detail below). The die (with the numbers one, two and three marked on opposite faces) is either a large one which can be rolled on the floor (a cube of foam with dots or numbers marked on it with felt pen) or a small wooden cube thrown in a plastic tray.

The first player rolls the die and moves forward the appropriate number of spaces. She then carries out the activity indicated. If she doesn't want to do the particular activity, she can 'pass', give the die to the next player and miss her next turn. The activities are:

1. Sing: the player either sings part of a song, with props if required, or a clip is played from the 'song' cassette and the player must guess who the singer is. The song cassette has several clips from different songs.
2. Create: the player takes some newspaper from the centre of the board and makes something from it (e.g. a hat).
3. Name game: the player rolls a ball to another player, saying her name. Other name games can also be used.
4. Dance: the player does a dance, or a movement, using props if she wishes (e.g. fan, scarf). The 'dance' cassette contains clips of various types of music which the player may wish to use.
5. Musical sound: the player makes a musical sound, using any of the musical instruments in the props. Alternatively, a clip from the 'musical sound' cassette (different musical instruments) is played and the player

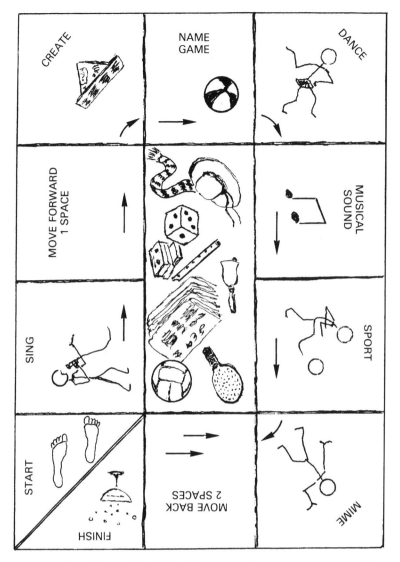

guesses what it is or identifies the correct instrument among the props.

6. Sport: the player acts out a sport, using the props.
7. Mime: any mime can be done and the other players guess what it is.

The game can be extended by using quiz cards for the 'Sing', 'Dance', 'Musical sound' and 'Sport' spaces. The player can choose to answer a question instead of doing the activities described above.

The Experiential Box (US in a BUS)

This is a game for a small group of people of any ability; it can be adapted for all and Janet and Marianne have found it a particularly good way of involving people who often find it difficult to contribute to a group activity.

107

The basic equipment is a box containing an assortment of objects. It helps if the box is a plastic one with open mesh sides, so that things in the box can be easily seen. All sorts of objects may be used:

- Piece of ridged plastic tubing
- Wine bag
- Koosh ball
- Plastic footpump (for inflating lilos)
- Silky scarf
- Small ball
- Square of strong plastic foam (sold in garden centres as a kneeling mat)

Each player takes a turn at picking one item from the box (there can be some creative interpretation of eye pointing for people who are at first reluctant or unable to choose). The player is then encouraged to do something with the object she has chosen. The object is passed round the group and then returned to the box. There isn't a 'wrong' way to use anything in the box, so nobody can fail at this game; even if someone simply drops their object, this can be copied and developed by the other members of the group.

For example, if the player chooses a Koosh ball and drops it, the next person can pick it up, lift it higher and drop it in an exaggerated way. The piece of tubing can be dragged over the arm of a wheelchair to make a noise, then passed to the next person who can make a different noise with it.

There is a seemingly endless variety of very simple things to be done with the objects and, as only one person is doing something at one time, it is a surprisingly effective way of making people more aware of each other. Because there is no pressure to do something in a particular way, nobody seems to be made anxious by this activity. Even just passing the chosen object to the next person is a contribution to the success of the game. The size of the group, the number of objects and the complexity of the game are all adaptable.

Chain and Slinky (US in a BUS)

This is another game devised by Marianne and Janet. You will need a plastic two-coloured Slinky and a length of chain (about 3 m of smooth linked chain). Double the chain and thread it straight through the Slinky. The loose ends and the Slinky are then held by one person ('the holder') and the other end is either held by the 'watcher', or linked over the handle of the watcher's wheelchair or another convenient anchorage point at eye level. The Slinky can then be released gradually by the holder.

The way the Slinky is released can be varied, depending on the watcher's wishes and the level of her involvement. For example, if you are introducing this game to a fairly quiet, withdrawn person it can be done gently, in stages with the holder retaining one end and giving a simple running commentary. Thus the watcher gets a quiet gentle view of changing colours, enhanced if the holder moves the chain slowly from side to side.

This can be made into an anticipation game, encouraging the watcher or other participants to join in the 'Ready Steady Go' business (part of the Slinky can be released with each word, ending with the whole Slinky on 'Go').

For some watchers, who are ready for it, it can be a noisy game with a surprise element — letting go of the whole Slinky at once and sending it crashing against the watcher's wheelchair handle at eye and ear level, or encouraging the watcher to reach out and rock the chain with the Slinky suspended on it.

A variation of the game is for two people to hold the ends of the chain (still threaded through the Slinky) and take it in turns to stand up/sit down or raise/lower their arms, sending the Slinky from one end to the other. Again, with two people holding an end each, the chain can be swung or waved (making sure that onlookers are out of range), whilst the Slinky rattles about on it. This is often accompanied by noise and laughter, especially when someone lets go inadvertantly.

Other DIY ideas include:

1. Make matching card games: this is most effective if you use photographs of objects or people familiar to the players. Take the photographs against a plain background which provides a good colour contrast between the object or person and the background. Look at local photographic services to see if they are offering a second set of prints free or at a cheap rate. Otherwise, send your films to Tripleprint (Freepost, Barnet, Herts EN5 1BR; Tel 081-953 9911) and you will get two small photographs with each standard one. Mount the photographs on pieces of thick card using spray mount, and cut the card with a craft knife on a plastic chopping board. Or you can mount them on pieces of hardboard, which will make them stronger and easier to pick up. Cut the hardboard to size, using a jigsaw or a bandsaw (if you have access to one). Stick each photograph to the rough side of the hardboard using PVA glue. In either case, cover the whole thing with self-adhesive clear plastic to protect it.
2. Make target games: sew coloured circles of fabric onto a large piece of material. You could give each circle a different points score, or do colour matching (red bean-bag on red circle, and so on). Sew concentric circles of fabric together, or mark concentric circles on an old sheet using fabric paints. Use with beanbags or Koosh balls.
3. Use the large, strong cardboard tubes from carpet shops for rolling ball games.
4. Make an obstacle course: under a table (with a blanket draped over the sides), through a streamer curtain, or plastic bottles hanging from the ceiling, or a doorway, over a mattress, under a parachute, and so on.

Commercial Equipment

Active Games

One of the most important items for game playing is a really good collection of balls. If you have a variety of types and sizes, and a bit of imagination, you need never be stuck for an instant activity. Balls can be used for:

1. Sensory stimulation (a range of textures, sounds, smells).
2. Target games — throwing a ball into a plastic bowl, a metal bucket or a cardboard box produces different sounds.
3. A game of human skittles (using a large inflated ball) — when hit, the 'skittles' can fall over with great dramatic action and noise !
4. Passing and rolling to each other, then for throwing and catching.
5. Hide and seek games.
6. Giant 'table skittles': place a foam football in a string bag and hang it from the ceiling. Swing the ball to knock over large skittles — either plastic sweet jars or lengths of cardboard tube from a roll of carpet. These tubes are very sturdy, about 10 cm diameter, with thick 'walls' (use a saw to cut them up).
7. The hanging football described above can also be used for kicking or hitting with a wooden bat. It should be used under supervision in case the player becomes tangled in the cord or rope suspending the ball.

The uses of Koosh balls are described separately, below, because they are so different from other balls.

The Koosh ball consists of a bundle of rubber filaments which are energy absorbing so that the ball doesn't bounce or roll, it won't hurt if it hits you, and it is easy to catch. The standard size is widely available in toy shops; the large size — called the Mondo Koosh — is available from Sportime and Mike Ayres & Co.

Koosh balls have so many uses:

1. Feel the texture and movement, stroke and tickle someone with it (a few people do not like the texture, but that is very unusual).
2. Look at a collection of Koosh — they come in various combinations of colours (some with better visual contrast than others) and some are fluorescent.
3. Hang the Koosh up, to swing and hit at. You can either attach a piece of strong elastic or cord to the loop on the ball, or you can buy a Yo-Koosh (from toy shops) which has elastic fitted.
4. Balance a Koosh on your head, or the back of your hand.
5. Make a target game by throwing the balls into hoops on the ground; smaller hoops will be more difficult.
6. Throw them at human targets, either stationary or moving.
7. Hit balls to each other using wooden bats (the type sold for beach games). Wrap foam plastic round the handles to make them more comfortable and easier to hold.

8. Throw Koosh balls at a football, to make it move. Try to make it move in a particular direction — quite difficult!

9. Throw a Koosh at a large inflated ball and it will bounce off at different angles (an idea developed by US in a BUS, see chapter 10).

10. Catch the Koosh in a plastic sieve, remove it and throw it back. With practice it is possible to throw the ball using the sieve.

11. Two (or more) people can toss a Koosh by holding the edges of a large towel or piece of material and pulling it taut so that the ball shoots in the air. Two teams, each with a piece of material, can toss the Koosh backwards and forwards between them.

12. Koosh balls can be used as an introduction to the game of Boccia (see below), or for practice when a competition set of Boccia balls is not available.

13. 'Hole in one' — players move round the room or garden, trying to throw the Koosh into a variety of containers. If you wish, you can develop a scoring system — two points for success at the first attempt, one for a second attempt, for example. Containers could be a washing-up bowl on a chair, a bucket on the ground, an ice-cream container floating in a large basin or tray of water, a small bowl with a hoop round it (standard points if the Koosh lands within the hoop, double points if it goes in the bowl).

Examples of other commercially available balls for your collection are:

1. Large clear PVC balls, some with small plastic balls inside (Mike Ayres & Co., Rompa): inflate them using a handblower (available from the same companies) or a cylinder vacuum cleaner (switch it to 'blow' for a few moments before you start to inflate the ball, to get rid of any dust in the pipes).

2. SloMo balls (Sportime): two sizes, move fairly slowly and can be inflated to varying degrees so that they are easier to hold and catch.

3. Soft Punch Ball (Rompa): similar to SloMo but only available in small size.

4. Balsac Balloon Ball (toy shops and Rompa): a large balloon is blown up inside a thin cotton bag. This produces a very light ball which will bounce and move slowly.

5. Knobbly Ball (Mike Ayres & Co., Rompa): a ball with bumps.

6. Hedgehog Ball (Mike Ayres & Co.), Spiky Ball (Rompa): a smaller ball with plastic spikes.

7. Noisy Ball (Rompa), Sounding Ball (TFH): ball with battery-powered bleeper.

8. Impossiball: the original version is hard to find now, but look for balls which are weighted on one side so that they roll in unexpected ways.

9. Snooker or pool balls: smooth, shiny and heavy; make an interesting noise as they roll and hit each other.

10. Carpet Bowls (sport shops): make a good noise as they roll on a hard surface and the bias makes them move in an interesting way.

11. Sqwish balls (toy shops): a heavy gell in a silky cover, a fascinating combination.
12. Gamester balls (educational catalogues): hollow plastic balls with holes; very light, about the size of a tennis ball, good for hanging up and threading on a rope.
13. Practice golf balls (sport shops): same as Gamester balls but smaller.
14. Table tennis balls (sport shops): especially the fluorescent ones.
15. Cat balls (pet shops): either plastic with a bell, or a metal 'cage' with a fluffy ball and a bell inside.
16. Bubbleheads (toy shops): small, clear plastic ball with another ball floating inside which stays still as the outer ball spins.
17. Patchwork balls (craft shops): add a different smell to each one (using food essences or essential oils) and remember to store them separately so that the smells don't mix. You could also make your own balls using different textures (craft books give patterns for patchwork balls).

Frisbees can also be used for various games, but the hard plastic ones are difficult to catch and hurt if they hit you! Flexible frisbees are better, and offer a range of interesting textures:

1. Flexible Frisbees (New Games UK): made of ripstop nylon, edged with the type of weighting that you find in shower curtains. They are easy to throw and catch and make a rustling sound when they are handled.
2. Sqwish Dish (toy shops): made by the manufacturers of the Sqwish ball, the dish is made of the same silky fabric with a rim of the gell. It flies like a frisbee but it is also excellent for passing games, in place of a quoit.
3. Woosh (toy shops, Rompa): made by the Koosh people, this consists of a wire rim with a band of nylon fabric stretched round it. Easy to hold and very light.

Various active social games are available:

1. Lawn Darts (Sportime): large plastic darts with rounded ends, rather than points. The object of the game is to throw them into the hoop provided. Similar games are available from some sport shops.
2. Lawn Horseshoes (Sportime): rubber horseshoes are thrown at a stake. This set is excellent because indoor mats are provided as well as the stakes for playing on grass.
3. Scatch/Supercatch (from NES Arnold and toy shops): two Velcro covered catch pads and a fluffy tennis ball. Each player catches the ball on the Velcro pad, removes it and throws it back. Good fun (plus the lovely noise of Velcro) but there is some criticism that Scatch does not encourage the catching action. When you catch a ball your hands move back towards your body, with Scatch you will probably move the pad forward to meet the ball. Velcro catching gloves are available (from some toy shops and TFH) which avoid this problem.
4. Boccia: this is a game which can be played by anyone, anywhere, at any level. It can be enjoyed as a social game but it is also played at

international competition level by disabled sportspeople. The aim is to get your balls as close to the target ball as possible. The balls may be thrown, kicked or rolled down a ramp. Boccia can be played by two players or by two teams of three players. The sets of leather-covered balls (six red, six blue and one white target ball) are available from Newton Products (see chapter 11). Further information and details of training courses are available from The National Boccia Association (see chapter 11).

5. Dartmaster Dartboard (from toy shops), Striker Dartboard (Sportime): two very similar pieces of equipment. The dartboard consists of rows of plastic 'spikes' and the darts (with weighted ends, but not points) stick in the board by fitting between the spikes. The dartboard can be used in the traditional way, or laid flat on the floor and the darts dropped onto it.

6. Rink Games (Rink Products): a range of large indoor social games which includes Rink (an ice hockey game), Snukatelle (in which discs are 'potted' using a cue), Rolladisc (plastic discs are rolled down a chute) and Rollaball (plastic balls are rolled into holes in the board). I find that the balls for this last game are too light for some people, and hard to control. Using carpet bowls instead provides more weight, an interesting noise and the bias sometimes helps the balls to go into the holes.

7. Supro Ice Hockey Game (Rompa): this item is expensive but it is a very sturdy version of the traditional game and it can be enjoyed by people with a wide range of abilities. It consists of a strong metal box with a clear cover. Each player/goal minder is controlled by a knob, which can be replaced by various handles to suit the person who is playing. A marble is inserted through a hole in the cover and reappears when a goal is scored.

8. Karom or Carrom (Karum's Workshop): large, wooden board game of Indian Snooker. The wooden playing pieces are potted by flicking them with a finger.

9. Table skittles: various versions are available in some of the rehab catalogues and at craft fairs. Woodworking books often given designs for them also. The basic idea is that the wooden skittles are knocked down by a ball swinging from a pole. What is needed is the old-fashioned version where all the skittles could be set upright again by pulling a lever or knob. This would make the game accessible to many more people, but I haven't seen them for many years.

Table Top Games

Some of the following games are designed for children but I believe that they may be used and enjoyed by adults — you may disagree.

1. Shapes Game (Galt): players move across the board according to the shapes indicated on the dice. Excellent game for all ages.
2. Pass the Bag (Child's Play): players distinguish wooden pieces by touch

and place them on their playing boards. Suitable game for adults, provided you throw the box away (childish illustrations).

3. Snail's Race Game (Ravensburger — from Raven and some toy shops): non-competitive race game. If you feel the bright colours and illustrations on the playing board are inappropriate, consider making Irma Mullin's version (see above).

4. Market Day (Ravensburger - from Raven and some toy shops): an enjoyable game with rules which are easy to understand e.g. if the square you have landed on shows two pigs you receive two pig cards.

5. Picture Lotto: most lotto games have unacceptable illustrations but Animal Lotto (Child's Play) has attractive drawings and Baby Animal Lotto (Ravensburger — from NES Arnold and some toy shops) uses photographs.

6. Dominoes: Geometric Tactile Dominoes (NES Arnold) are large wooden dominoes with raised shapes. Giant Finger Touch Dominoes (TFH) are large, with raised coloured spots (1 to 6). Commercial texture dominoes never give a large enough piece of texture to touch and it is better to make your own, by sticking textures to pieces of wood or cardboard. You can make picture dominoes using appropriate pictures cut out of catalogues, or photographs (see 'Matching Cards' in the DIY section, above, for a description of the techniques involved).

7. RNIB Games: the Royal National Institute for the Blind supply various games for visually impaired people, such as board games with playing pieces which are distinguishable by shape as well as colour, and adaptations of popular games such as Connect 4.

8. Colour Board Game (Rompa): this is a large version of Ludo. The large wooden board has recessed holes into which the chunky wooden playing pieces fit. Other games used to be available in the same range and they occasionally reappear in the educational catalogues. They are worth looking out for, as the wooden pieces are easy to hold and the recessed holes provide stability.

9. Dice: wooden dice with 1 to 6 dots, approximately 3 cm in size, are available from many of the catalogues. Larger plastic or foam dice with dots are available from Winslow Press and from NES Arnold. The latter also sell large dice with colours or numbers and a set consisting of a die with raised shapes on it and a pack of counters in the same shapes, so that you can make up your own games.

10. Social Skills games: The Consortium produces an excellent range of games and related materials for people with learning disabilities, including:

    ● Bus Ride: a photographic guide to making a bus journey, which may be used in conjunction with 'On the Road'
    ● On the Road: a travel skills board game.
    ● Starfoods: a shopping game

    All the materials are produced to a very high standard, with clear photographs, cassettes with appropriate songs, users' handbooks, and so on.

Adapted Games

The Meldreth Series

This series of adapted sports activities for people with severe disabilities was devised by Len Reed at Meldreth Manor School in Cambridgeshire. Len has devised adaptations for bowls (using unbiased Scottish carpet bowls), ten-pin bowling, billiards, cricket, snooker and tennis. Each game may be played at various skill levels, each with its own set of rules.

I particularly like the scoreboard which Len devised for many of his games: rectangular pieces of plywood of different colours and heights (proportional to the points score they represent) are slotted into a board. This visual representation of the score is much more relevant for the players and the idea could be used in many other games.

Books describing the principles of the games, the specifications for equipment and the rules are available; there is also a video showing the games being played (see chapter 11). Occasional training events are organized — for further information, contact Pro-Motion (see chapter 10).

Nottingham Polytechnic Adapted Games

Various activities, games and sports have been adapted by Doug Williamson and his colleagues to enable people with disabilities to take part in physical recreation. Games include Floor Snooker, Table Bowls, and Polybat — an excellent version of table tennis in which the bat is in contact with the table and is used to push the ball. The game can be played with a Gamester ball or practice golfball but it can be slowed down even more by using a hedgehog ball. There is also a design for a metal ramp which can be used as an assistive device for ten-pin bowling.

The games and equipment are described in a Workshop Manual which is available from Doug Williamson (see chapter 11).

Co-operative Games

These are alternatives to traditional competitive games and they are particularly suitable for groups of people (children or adults) with a wide range of abilities. The games involve very little equipment and they can cater for large or small groups. Many of the activities involve touch and close physical contact, which makes them especially beneficial but also possibly threatening until people get used to the idea. Some of the games will need adapting to suit the understanding and mobility of the group.

There are several books on co-operative games (see chapter 11) and there is a video by Mildred Masheder which explains the principles of the games and shows children playing them. However, the best way to learn is by experience. Many playworkers and adventure playground staff use co-operative games — you could contact them (through your local authority leisure or recreation department) and ask if you could visit and learn from them.

New Games UK organize training courses which are a good learning opportunity, and also a chance to meet people who are using the games in various settings.

Parachute Games

There can be few pieces of leisure equipment which are as versatile, portable and easy to store as a parachute. They are expensive to buy, but they are a very worthwhile investment as they can be used for boisterous active games, quiet relaxation, music and movement activities and drama, and they can also be used to transform the environment (see chapter 5).

It is still possible to obtain parachutes from the RAF or the US Air Force, but it is becoming increasingly difficult because so many people are trying to get them! However, the parachutes have to be disposed of after a certain number of jumps, so contact the person in charge of the stores at your nearest airbase. Personnel parachutes are light and silky, but probably won't be very exciting colours. Cargo parachutes are much heavier — you won't be able to use them for games, but they may be OK for drama or for creating a circus tent.

If you are unable to find a free one, parachutes (or, more accurately, play canopies) are available from several catalogues. Quality varies a great deal however. Sportime supply a range of sizes of parachutes, with storage bags, which are excellent. Flying Objects supply a set consisting of a 5 m diameter parachute and bag, two books and a video on co-operative games and a games reminder sheet, at a very reasonable price (see chapter 11).

Before starting the games, players should remove any sharp jewellery, hair ornaments, buckles, etc. which might injure people or damage the parachute. If you are playing indoors, check that there are no nails or other objects in the walls or ceiling on which the parachute might snag. It is important to check the parachute regularly for small holes or stitching which is coming undone and to repair it promptly before the damage can get worse.

People who use wheelchairs will need enablers for some of the games, unless they can propel themselves. Remember also that players who use wheelchairs will be unable to reach up as far as people who are standing. It may be advisable to have everyone seated for some of the games which involve raising the parachute.

Players often get very excited and involved in the games and grip the parachute much harder than they need to. In between games, ask everyone to relax their hands and move their fingers on the silky material (I call it 'playing the piano').

Here are a few examples of games and activities you can do:

1. Mushrooming: do this as a starter game, to get everyone in the mood and used to the parachute. The players are evenly spaced around the

edge of the parachute, they gently raise the parachute as far as it will go and then lower it. Repeat this a few times. If everyone takes a step towards the centre as the parachute is raised, it will go much higher. You can use this as a closing activity as well. In this case, ask everyone to let go when you say 'Go'. Wait until the parachute is reaching its highest point before saying the word. The parachute will drift down gently and everyone should feel very peaceful.

2. Billowing: two or three people lie in the middle of the parachute and the remaining players gently billow the parachute around them. Place a thin mat under the parachute, for comfort, unless there is carpet on the floor.

3. Ball down the hole: most parachutes have a small hole in the centre. Divide the players into two colour teams, positioned alternately around the parachute. Each team has a small ball in their colour and tries to be the first to get their ball down the hole, by bouncing or rolling the ball on the parachute.

4. Popcorn: collect a large number of foam and plastic balls (not too heavy) and place them on the parachute. The players try to set them all bouncing (like popcorn in a pan) and then, when the leader gives the word, bounce them all off the parachute as quickly as possible.

5. Waves: demonstrate to the players how to create a wave around the edge of the parachute by alternately lowering and raising each hand. Place a large soft ball (a SloMo ball is ideal) on the edge of the parachute and let the wave action move it round the circle. Change direction.

6. Name Swap: the players raise and lower the parachute. When it is low, the leader says 'John swap with Zia' (choosing players who are roughly opposite each other). As the parachute is raised, the named players move under it and swap places. This continues, with other people being named and different players taking it in turns to be leader. The same game can be played using colours or items of clothing instead of names, e.g. everyone wearing blue (or wearing a jumper) swap over.

7. Air conditioning: two or three players lie on the floor under the parachute. The remaining players gently lower the parachute onto them, move it from side to side (to give them a 'tickle') and then slowly raise it again. The movements should be gentle so that the air currents created are a breeze, not a gale!

8. Squash: spread the parachute out over mats or a soft carpet. Blow air under it, using a handblower or a cylinder vacuum cleaner. The players kneel, crawl and roll on the parachute to try to squash it flat.

9. Swaying: one person lies in the centre of the parachute. The players roll up the edge of the circle until the fabric is taut then, lifting towards the waist (no higher, to avoid back strain), raise the person off the ground and sway the parachute gently from side to side. Never toss someone in a parachute — you risk injury to the person and the other players and damage to the parachute.

10. Dancing: choose some rhythmic, lively music (such as folk or country dancing music). Sit in a circle, holding the parachute. When the music starts, pass the parachute round in time to the music, reversing the direction occasionally. You can also dance by holding the parachute and

the players moving round in a circle, changing direction, moving into the centre and out again.

Outdoors

Many of the games already described in this chapter may be played outdoors or indoors, but this section is about activities which are most likely to be done outside.

Many leisure facilities are becoming more accessible to people with disabilities. Nature trails, bird sanctuaries, woodland and downland can all be enjoyed for their own sake but can also be the setting for impromptu games — finding (but not picking) flowers, spotting different types of birds or butterflies, throwing pebbles into a pond or stream (not if there are fish), matching fallen leaves, and so on. And then there is Poohsticks — one of the best games ever invented! Take some short lengths of different coloured wool with you and find a bridge over a stream which is flowing steadily, but not too fast. Each player finds a small twig and ties their colour of wool to it. The players line up on the upstream side of the bridge, drop their twigs in the water, move to the downstream side and wait. The winner is the player whose twig appears first.

Kite flying is another popular pastime. There are specialist kite shops in many areas (look in Yellow Pages) and kites are also available from some of the special needs suppliers:

- Sled Kite (Rompa)
- Ram Kite (Rompa)
- Ferrari Kite (Mike Ayres & Co.)
- Windsock (Rompa)

Brookite sell a wide range of kites and windsocks, plus materials for making them.

You can make your own kites (see books in chapter 11) from paper, polythene, or from ripstop nylon (available from kite shops and by mail order from Brookite).

It is never easy to find large activity equipment which is adult-sized but there are some useful items:

1. Adult Swing Seat (TFH): a large support seat with a pommel and straps. One leisure library uses this in conjunction with large foam blocks, to encourage leg movements to knock them down.
2. Coracle (TFH): a swingboat which the person can lie in.
3. Giant Top (TFH)/Roll and Spin Top (Mike Ayres & Co.)/ Spinning Saucer (Rompa): this shallow fibreglass bowl is big enough (80 cm diameter) for some adults to sit in it and rock or spin, but two leisure libraries also reported that their customers enjoyed spinning balls and other objects in the bowl.
4. Side by Side Cycle (Mike Ayres & Co.): two people can cycle together.

5. The Duet (Neatwork): this vehicle consists of the back of a conventional cycle with a wheelchair at the front which is slightly tilted back, so that it runs on its rear wheels. The wheelchair can be detached when you arrive at your destination.

Further advice on tricycles and bicycles may be obtained from the Disabled Living Foundation (see chapter 10).

9

What Can I Do With ...?

Although it is usually best to start by considering the person and deciding what equipment to make, it is sometimes helpful to look at the materials you have and think what to do with them.

This chapter looks at some items which may be lying around and suggests some ideas for using them — I'm sure you can suggest plenty more !

Paper Bags

1. Sort acorns, conkers, buttons, etc. into different bags — or red things, blue things.
2. Make an instant feelie bag: put differently shaped and textured objects into a large bag, put your hands in and try to identify the objects.
3. Use large paper carrier bags or grocery sacks to make masks. Cut eye holes, decorate with felt pens or paint.
4. Use small bags as hand puppets. Twist corners into 'ears' and draw an animal face.
5. Some stationers use very attractive patterned paper bags; tear the bags into small pieces and use to make collage pictures.
6. Crumple bags into balls and use for various games — throwing into a box, through a hoop, etc.
7. Sort the bags according to size, fit them inside each other, how many times do we have to fold this large bag before it will fit inside the small bag?
8. Fold bags into various shapes (a book on Origami will give you some ideas). If you use coloured and patterned bags, the folded shapes could be hung up as a mobile.

Cardboard Boxes

1. Collect various sizes of boxes, tape the ends closed, build a skyscraper or a wall, then knock it down.
2. Tear them up, then collect up all the pieces and take them to a recycling point.

3. Make giant sculptures, using boxes of various shapes, cardboard tubes, etc.
4. Paint them — painting a three-dimensional shape is a very different experience from painting on paper.
5. See how many boxes you can fit inside each other.
6. Throw balls or sock sponges (see below) into a box. Someone can hold the box and move it to make it easier (or harder!) to get them in.
7. Reinforce a large box with extra pieces of cardboard and use it for light stimulation work (see chapter 4).
8. Cut different shaped holes in the sides of a large box (using a craft knife with care). Cover each hole with a different colour of acetate or cellophane. Lie inside the box and look out through the windows. Shine sunlight or lamplight through the windows.
9. Make a 'graffiti block'. Find a large, sturdy box, tape the ends closed and paint the whole thing with white emulsion. When the paint is dry, give everyone large felt pens so that they can cover the box with names, drawings, squiggles, etc.
10. Make a sorting game — one box for balls, another for cushions, another for balloons, and so on. Spread them around the room to encourage movement.
11. Stuff each box firmly with crumpled newspaper, especially the edges and corners. Then wash hands to remove the ink! Tape each box closed. Decorate with powder paint mixed with PVA glue and a little water, to produce a hard wearing, shiny finish. These adult-sized building blocks will last quite a long time, if they have been well stuffed.
12. Cut out large shapes (trees, cacti, etc.), paint them and add them to murals. Remember that corrugated cardboard, because of the way it is made, bends in one direction and is very stiff in others.

Plastic Bottles

Collect a wide range of plastic bottles: transparent soft-drink bottles (from the small size through to 2 litre ones), cosmetics and shampoo bottles in different sizes and colours, fabric conditioner bottles with handles, and so on. Choose the right sort of bottle for the person who is going to use it — tough guys may need a sturdy fabric conditioner bottle, gentler people can use the flimsier drinks bottles.

Make sure that the bottles are completely clean (particularly important if you are using bottles which have contained detergents or fabric conditioner). Soak the bottles to remove the labels (a few labels peel off, but most will need soaking). It is very difficult to completely remove all the glue on some bottles, and most solvents will attack the plastic. If you are going to fill bottles with dry materials, leave them in an airing cupboard for several days to make sure that they are completely dry.

You will need to experiment to find which glue is suitable for sticking the cap on the bottle. Bostik or UHU are okay for some plastics, but will dissolve others. Polystyrene cement (sold for model making) is usually all right. You can secure the cap with PVC tape (after the glue has dried), to make it even safer.

1. Fillings for bottles:
   - Sequins in a small bottle.
   - Dried peas, lentils, lengths of spaghetti (never use dried beans if there is the slightest danger of people getting at the contents, as some types can cause a nasty stomach upset if swallowed raw).
   - Water, glitter and glycerine (available from chemists or cake-decorating shops, makes the water thicker and holds the glitter in suspension better).
   - Coloured water and metallic buttons — try blue water and silver buttons, red water and gilt buttons.
   - Water and floating fluorescent table-tennis balls (from sports shops and departments) in a wide-necked bottle or plastic sweet jar.
   - Silver sand and coloured glitter.
2. Make a sound-matching game. Collect several identical opaque bottles and put the same filling in pairs of the bottles (e.g. sand, lentils, dried peas, bells, marbles).
3. Buy a Tornado Tube from TFH. Use this to connect two large drinks bottles (one containing some water) together. Turning the bottles over produces a whirlpool effect as the water runs through. You can make the effect more spectacular by adding glycerine and silver glitter to the water and shining a light on the bottles.
4. Take two 1 litre bottles and a 30 cm length of clear plastic tubing (available from wine-making and aquarium shops). Choose a diameter of tubing which will just fit over the neck of the bottle. Place some water, food colouring and washing-up liquid in one of the bottles and, keeping it upright, glue each end of the tubing over the neck of one of the bottles. Once the glue is dry, you have a visually stimulating object which encourages large movements as the water is tipped from one bottle to the other.

5. ### *Egg Timer*

This design is from 'Make It Simple' by Carol Ouvry and Suzie Mitchell (1990, The Consortium) and is included here by kind permission of the authors.

This item provides interesting visual effects linked with sound. Take two small drinks bottles and a short length of plastic tubing (just long enough to fit over the necks of the two bottles). Place sand, beads, buttons, or some other filling in one of the bottles. Smear polystyrene cement round the neck of the filled bottle and the inside of one end of the tube. Place the tube over the neck of the bottle and hold in place until the glue is dry. Repeat with the other end of the tube and the other (empty) bottle.

6. *Spinning Bottles (JD)*

Collect several cylindrical bottles (cosmetics, shampoo, bubble bath). Drill through each bottle, from side to side, making a hole which is large enough for a piece of dowel to pass through. You will find it easier to use a small drill first, so that the hole acts as a guide for the larger drill. The bottles should turn easily on the dowel but the holes should not be so large that the filling can escape.

Place a different sound in each bottle — bell, dried peas, lentils, metal washers, etc. — and glue the top on. Paint the bottles with enamel paint or decorate them with coloured labels, PVC tape, or scraps of Fablon.

Thread the bottles onto the dowel, with a short length of plastic tubing between each bottle as a spacer. The dowel can be suspended from an existing frame, if you have one, or you can make a wooden stand for it.

Wine Bags

It is amazing, but some people still don't realize that inside those cardboard wine boxes you see in supermarkets and off-licences there are the most wonderful plasticized foil bags. Collecting them could not be easier — you can nobly volunteer to drink the wine! However, if you want a large number of bags it might be advisable to get other people involved. Ask local social clubs, student unions and pubs if they use them. Catering firms often use them for big functions (they sometimes have larger wine boxes). Ask your local off-licence if you could put a notice by the display of wine boxes, asking customers to save the bags.

When you have your bags, rinse them by holding the open valve upside down under a running tap, slosh the water around and squeeze it out. Repeat this a few times, but don't worry too much — the smell of the wine is part of the fun of using these bags and it takes a very long time before the wine starts to smell unpleasantly 'off'.

1. Inflate the bag and hang it (by the valve) where it will catch the light and people can watch the reflections as it spins.
2. Before inflating, smooth the bag flat and make sure the outside is dry. Stick self-adhesive diffraction foil on both sides of the bag (using different colours or patterns of foil if you want to). Inflate the bag and hang up as above.
3. Partially inflate the bag and scrunch it between your hands.
4. Put some water in the bag and partially inflate it. Moving the bag makes a lovely sloshing sound. Put the bag in the fridge for a while, to make the water cold. Run warm water into the bag for a different sensation.
5. This idea comes from US in a BUS (see chapter 10). Partially inflate the bag and place it on the person's lap or wheelchair tray. Place a Koosh ball on one end of the bag. When she drops her hand on the other end of the bag, the Koosh will fly off, thus producing a big effect from a small movement. This can be extended into an anticipation game, followed by

123

searching for the ball. It can include other people and can even be turned into a competition (how far can you send the ball, can you make it jump over a chair, guess the direction, and so on), depending on the players' abilities.

6. Have 'pillow fights' with the inflated bags (holding the valve).

7. Hang up the inflated bag to be punched or kicked. Hanging the bag by the valve is the easiest way of suspending it, but it also means that people are unlikely to be hit by the valve.

8. Inflate the bag completely and place it on the floor. Throw Koosh balls or sponge socks (see below) at the bag to make it move.

9. Collect a large number of wine bags and make sure that the outside surfaces are clean and dry. Stick small pieces of self-adhesive Velcro in several places on each side of each bag, making sure that the 'hook' and 'loop' pieces are evenly distributed. Inflate the bags and attach them together to form giant sculptures.

10. Collect a large number of bags and flatten them out. Sew them together, through the edges (obviously making sure that you don't puncture the bags themselves), using carpet twine (a strong linen thread sold in haberdashers). Make sure that all the valves are on the same side of this mat you are forming, so that they can be on the underside when the mat is in use. Inflate the bags different amounts and use it to feel and to lie on.

11. And finally, when you have exhausted all the other possibilities, cut up the bags and use them for art work or mobiles!

Socks

You can make various items of leisure equipment from socks and it is a good way of using up the odd socks that everyone seems to have! Don't be tempted to use very old and worn socks — they will not be strong enough. Socks can usually be bought very cheaply from market stalls and seconds shops.

1. Make instant feelie bags: put different textures in each ankle sock (dried peas, lentils, rice, buttons, polystyrene packing shapes) and sew up the end of the sock. Provide a plastic bowl as a container so that the socks can be taken out, explored and put back.

2. Sock sponges are easy to grasp and can be used for target games (throwing at skittles, or into a box or a hoop on the floor). More importantly they can simply be used for letting off steam — throwing them around and collecting them up, throwing them at people, and so on. Use men's socks (because they are bigger than ankle socks but not as long as knee-high ones). Cut large rectangular bath sponges in half, lengthwise, using a pair of scissors with long blades or a serrated bread knife. Alternatively you could cut rectangles approximately 5 cm x 5 cm x 15 cm from a large piece of foam plastic.

Turn a sock inside out and place one of the sponges in the foot of the sock. Twist the sock round and double it back on itself, thus forming a

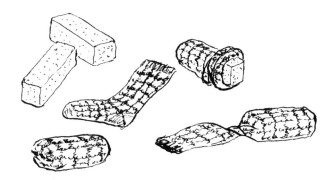

second layer over the sponge (the sock will now be right side out). Sew up the end of the sock. Repeat with the remaining socks and sponges.

3. Make a wall hanging. Collect together fluorescent and brightly-coloured socks. Fill them with various materials — polyester stuffing, tights cut up in small pieces, bubble plastic, polystyrene packing shapes, a plastic film canister containing some rice, bells, marbles, a flat plastic squeaker (from craft shops), a deflated metallic balloon or a piece of survival blanket (rustling noise), and so on. Arrange the socks on a piece of white or black fabric (whichever will give the best contrast with the socks you have chosen) and machine across the top of each sock twice (to keep the filling in place and to attach it to the fabric). Hang it on the wall, or place it on the floor or table to be explored.

The next two designs are from Touch Toys Inc., and they are included here by kind permission of Mrs Henriette Zegers Ten Horn, the Founder and President.

Touch Toys Inc., started in 1971, is an international group of women, living in the Washington DC area of the USA, dedicated to creating special toys for visually impaired and disabled children (see chapter 11).

I asked permission to include the Snake that Swallowed an Egg and the Caterpillar because I have used them with adults and found them very popular.

Snake that Swallowed an Egg

Take two knee-length socks. Use new, strong socks and this item will be very sturdy. Pull one sock over your arm, with your hand in the foot (as if you were going to darn it). Pull several (at least ten) cut-off legs of tights, one at a time, over your arm. Finally pull the second sock over the top. While all the layers are still on your arm take several stitches at the toes, through all the layers, using strong button thread.

Slide the sock/tights/sock off your arm carefully and sew firmly round the top of the socks and tights, making sure that you catch all the layers. Place a smooth rubber ball, slightly larger than the circumference of the sock, inside the inner sock. Sew the opening together, tucking the edges in neatly.

Sew two buttons (eyes) on the snake's head (the toe) and a forked tongue, cut from a piece of thin leather or PVC. The buttons are good to explore with the fingers (bearing in mind that this item may be enjoyed by people who cannot see it), but if you are worried about them, embroider eyes or sew on two small circles of felt.

The snake can be grasped, swung, pulled and the ball can be squeezed up and down its length.

Caterpillar

This is an adapted version of the Touch Toys design, to make it more suitable for the people we are considering in this book.

You will need a metal Slinky (one of those spirals which 'walk' down stairs) and a knee length sock. Place the Slinky inside the sock and close the end with strong thread and neat stitches. Stretching the toe of the sock over one end of the Slinky, oversew round the first circle of the spiral so that sock and Slinky are joined together. Repeat this process with the other end.

Make a large, wool pompom and attach it to one end, for the head of the caterpillar. Make or buy a tassle and attach it to the other end, for the tail.

The Caterpillar has an interesting texture, movement and noise. It is not as sturdy as the Snake, but being in a sock does protect the Slinky to a certain extent from being over-stretched or tangled.

Magnetic Tape

You can buy small quantities of magnetic tape (a flexible strip which acts as a magnet and is self-adhesive) from stationers and Tandy shops, but if you are going to use a lot it will be more economic to buy a large roll through the educational catalogues or the special needs suppliers. Mike Ayres & Co. and Rompa sell two widths (7.5 mm and 12.5 mm), TFH only sell the narrower width. Magnetic tape is expensive but the trick is to only use small pieces and to position them on the object where they will be most effective. For square or rectangular shapes, this will mean a small piece in each corner. Other shapes will probably be okay with three pieces evenly distributed, so that they don't wobble, but you may need a few more.

There is a possible source of free magnetic tape — the doors of most modern fridges and freezers have magnetic tape behind the rubber seal on the door or lid. Civic amenity sites usually keep old fridges and freezers separate from the rest of the rubbish — take a craft knife with you and ask the manager of the site if you can remove the magnetic strip. Refrigeration suppliers often take away the old model when they deliver a new fridge or freezer — you could approach them as well.

When you have made any of the items described below, you can use them on:

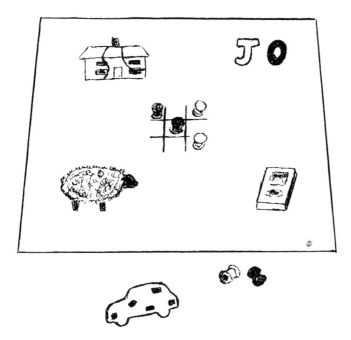

- the metal surface of a fridge, freezer, washing machine or tumble drier;
- a baking sheet;
- a small metal board (from educational catalogues) used horizontally on a table or wheelchair tray;
- a large metal board with a stand (from Rompa or TFH);
- the Magnetic Bookrest (from TFH), which is useful because the angle of the surface can be altered but the woodgrain effect does not provide a good contrast for many of the materials.

Here are some ideas for things to make using magnetic tape:

1. Collect small packets — jelly, stock cubes, variety packs of cereal, etc. Stuff them firmly with torn-up newspaper (especially the corners and edges) and tape them closed. Cover each packet completely with self-adhesive clear plastic and stick a small piece of magnetic tape in each corner of the back.
2. Buy wooden or plastic mosaic pieces, attach magnetic tape, and use for pattern making. You could make your own mosaic pieces from thin plywood, but the shapes must be cut accurately so that they fit together properly.
3. Attach magnetic tape to a set of dominoes (dot, picture or texture).
4. Buy sets of wooden templates (animals, vehicles, etc.) from toy shops or craft fairs. Paint houses, trees, vehicles appropriately. Stick textures — leather, suede, fleece, long and short pile fur fabric — on the animal templates using Copydex. Attach magnetic tape.
5. Sets of plywood letters, numbers or shapes can have texture added using Fablon green 'baize', self-adhesive Vivelle (a plush-coated craft material

in a range of colours, from Rompa) or Coversoft (similar product, from NES Arnold). Place the letters or numbers face down on the sticky surface and, resting them on a plastic chopping board, trim round each shape with the point of a sharp craft knife. Attach magnetic tape.

6. Stick self-adhesive diffraction foil onto plywood shapes, add magnetic tape, and use them on a black baking tray for good contrast.

7. Magnetic tape can also be used on wooden jigsaw pieces. The non-interlocking type can be pushed together on the board. Interlocking pieces will have to be picked up and fitted over each other. Make sure the pieces don't wobble (add extra pieces of magnetic tape if necessary) as this will make it more difficult to fit the pieces together.

8. Attach tape to coloured cotton reels (from educational catalogues) and use them as counters for games (marking the playing surface on a white metal board with felt pens) or for sorting and counting.

9. Magnetic tape can also be put on draughts or wooden noughts and crosses, and the appropriate playing board marked out.

10. Mount photographs of family and friends on plywood (using PVA glue) or thick card (using spray mount). Cover with self-adhesive clear plastic to protect them, if you wish, and attach magnetic tape. Arrange the photographs on a metal surface — you now have a 'photograph album' which can be looked at more easily than a book, and the photos can be moved around and grouped as desired.

10

Useful Organizations

ACTIVE

68 Churchway, London NW1 1LT; Tel 071 387 9592
This organization aims to help people with disabilities to lead more active and independent lives by sharing ideas on one-off pieces of equipment and modifications. Local ACTIVE groups design, make and modify equipment — often for play and leisure use. The national organization (part of the National Association of Toy and Leisure Libraries) publishes a series of worksheets giving instructions for making various living and leisure aids.

Disabled Living Foundation

380-384 Harrow Road, London W9 2HU; Tel 071 289 6111
Provides practical advice and information on all aspects of living with disability for disabled and elderly people and their carers. There is an enquiry service, staffed by therapists, and an equipment centre with a wide range of disability equipment on display. DLF publishes books, resource papers, advice notes and the Handbook — a comprehensive directory of daily living equipment.

Information Exchange

Wendy McCracken, Oakes Green, Royal Schools for the Deaf, Stanley Road, Cheadle Hulme, Cheshire SK8 6RF; Tel 061 437 6744
Not an organization, but a wonderful journal by and for parents and workers concerned with children and young people who have sensory impairments and other disabilities. Although aimed at younger age groups, much of the information is useful for people working in adult services.

National Association of Toy and Leisure Libraries

68 Churchway, London NW1 1LT; Tel 071 387 9592

Leisure libraries cater for adults and young people over 16 years of age with special needs due to learning or profound multiple disabilities. They lend leisure and recreation equipment and encourage hobbies and other interests. The Association can provide details of existing leisure libraries and advice on setting one up.

Planet

Save the Children, Cambridge House, Cambridge Grove, London W6 0LE; Tel 081 741 4054 (new address from April 1995)
Planet is a national information resource on play, leisure and recreation for children, young people and adults with disabilities. It provides advice on equipment, activities and organizations and has a resource centre which may be visited by appointment. The centre consists of a display room of equipment, a small multisensory room, and a reference library of books, journals and videos. Planet is a partnership project between Mencap, Save the Children and The Spastics Society.

Playtrac

c/o Horizon Trust Harperbury, Harper Lane, Radlett, Herts WD7 9HQ; Tel 0923 854861 ext 4385
Playtrac is a mobile training resource on play and leisure for people with learning disabilities. The service is funded through North West Thames Regional Health Authority and is free to staff from health, education and social services, parents and voluntary agencies within the Region. Playtrac works with staff teams and other groups, offering training and consultancy in the workplace. It also organizes regional training events and publishes leaflets on a range of play and leisure topics.

Pro-Motion

Recreation Services, Scope, 11 Churchill Park, Colwick, Nottingham NG4 2HE; Tel 0602 401202
Pro-Motion aims to develop sport and recreation opportunities for people with a severe physical or learning disability. It is a joint venture between Cerebral Palsy Sport and the United Kingdom Sports Association for People with a Mental Handicap. The project publishes a resource guide, organizes training courses and is setting up six resource bases around the country to gather and share information on equipment and activities.

RNIB Information Service on Multiple Disability

Gill Levy, RNIB, 224 Great Portland Street, London W1N 6AA; Tel 071 388 1266

The Service provides information and publishes leaflets and a newsletter to assist staff and carers of adults who have visual and learning disabilities or profound and multiple disabilities.

Scrapbanks

Scrapbanks, sometimes called play resource centres, collect surplus and waste materials from industry and commerce and make them available for use in play and creative activities by children's and special needs organizations. There are over forty resource centres around the country, most in urban areas. They usually charge an annual membership fee and member groups can make unlimited visits to collect materials for free or for a small charge. Contact the Federation of Resource Centres for details of your nearest resource centre: Federation of Resource Centres, 25 Bullivant Street, St Anne's, Nottingham NG3 4AT.

US in a BUS

The Royal Earlswood Hospital, Brighton Road, Redhill, Surrey RH1 6JL; Tel 0737 768511 ext 8260. This is a small mobile project operating in four Surrey hospitals. Its aim is to provide leisure/pleasure activities and experiences for adults with multiple and severe learning disabilities. Marianne Hecker and Janet Gurney, who started the project, have developed many simple and innovative ideas for interacting with people who are often isolated by the profound nature of their disabilities or by challenging behaviour.

11

Resources

Educational Suppliers

Child's Play (International)
Ashworth Road, Bridgemead, Swindon SN5 7YD
Tel: 0793 616286   Fax: 0793 512795

Hope Education
Orb Mill, Huddersfield Road, Waterhead, Oldham OL4 2ST
Tel: 061 633 6611   Fax: 061 633 3431

Galt Educational
Culvert Street, Oldham, Lancashire OL4 2ST
Tel: 061 627 5086   Fax: 061 627 1543

NES Arnold
Ludlow Hill Road, West Bridgford, Nottingham NG2 6HD
Tel: 0602 452201   Fax: 0602 452328

Raven Educational Supplies
13a Victoria Road, Wellingborough, Northants NN8 1HN
Tel: 0933 279108   Fax: 0933 229426

Specialist Suppliers

The Consortium — see Resources for Learning Difficulties

Edu-Play
Units H & I, Vulcan Business Centre, Vulcan Road, Leicester LE5 3EB
Tel: 0533 625827   Fax: 0533 625663

Mike Ayres Design
Unit 8, Shepherds Grove, Stanton, Bury St Edmunds, Suffolk IP31 2AR
Tel: 0359 251551   Fax: 0359 251707

Quest Enabling Designs (switches)
Ability House, 242 Gosport Road, Fareham, Hants PO16 0SS
Tel: 0329 828444

Resources for Learning Difficulties
The Consortium, Jack Tizard School, Finlay Street, London SW6 6HB
Tel: 071 736 8877

RNIB
Customer Services, PO Box 173, Peterborough PE2 6WS
Tel: 0345 023153

Rompa
Goyt Side Road, Chesterfield S40 2PH
Tel: 0246 211777   Fax: 0246 221802

TFH
76 Barracks Road, Sandy Lane Industrial Estate, Stourport-on-Severn DY13 9QB
Tel: 0299 827820   Fax: 0299 827035

Suppliers of Materials

Brookite (kite fabric)
Brightley Mill, Okehampton EX20 1RR
Tel: 0837 53315   Fax: 0837 53223

Edu-Play (diffraction foil, bells)
Units H & I, Vulcan Business Centre, Vulcan Road, Leicester LE5 3EB
Tel: 0533 625827   Fax: 0533 625663

Lakeland Plastics (drip dry carousel, net washing bags)
Alexandra Buildings, Windermere LA23 1BQ
Tel: 05394 88100

Making Leisure Equipment (chapter 2)

These books contain many designs which are suitable for adults:

Easy to Make Toys for Your Handicapped Child
Don Caston 1983 Souvenir Press

Make it Simple
Carol Ouvry and Suzie Mitchell 1990 The Consortium (Jack Tizard School, Finlay Street, London SW6 6HB

Play Helps
Roma Lear 1993 (third edition) Butterworth-Heinemann

More Play Helps
Roma Lear 1990 Butterworth-Heinemann

Working Wooden Toys
Marion Millett 1985 Blandford Press

Touch Toys and How to Make Them
Available from: Mrs Eleanor Timberg, Vice President, Touch Toys Inc.,
3519 Porter Street NW, Washington DC 20016, USA.

Sensory Stimulation (chapter 4)

The following companies supply 'gimmicky' items which are useful for a sensory bank:

Barnum's
67 Hammersmith Road, London W14 8UZ
Tel: 071 602 1211   Fax: 071 603 9945

Curiosity Shop
Admail 50, Leicester LE5 5DL
Tel: 0274 571611

Direct Choice UK
Euroway Business Park, Swindon SN5 8SN
Tel: 0793 513946

Frog Frolics
123 Ifield Road, London SW10 9AR
Tel: 071 370 4358   Fax: 071 370 6384

Innovations (Mail Order) Ltd/International Buyers Guide
Euroway Business Park, Swindon SN5 8SN
Tel: 0793 513946

Natural History Museum Collection
Euroway Business Park, Swindon, Wiltshire SN5 8SN
Tel: 0793 431900   Fax: 0793 485636

Science Museum Catalogue
Euroway Business Park, Swindon, Wiltshire SN5 8SN
Tel: 0793 480200   Fax: 0793 485636

Stockingfillas
Euroway Business Park, Blagrobe, Swindon SN5 8SN
Tel: 0793 513945

Tridias
124 Walcot Street, Bath BA1 5BG
Tel: 0225 469455 Fax: 0225 448592

Other companies mentioned in the chapter are:

SNC Playring (Pat Mat, Stim-Mobile, etc.)
53 Westbere Road, West Hampstead, London NW2 3SP
Tel/Fax: 071 794 9497

Tocki (glitter tubes)
Unit 9, Riverview Business Centre, Riverview Road, Beverley HU17 0LD
Tel: 0482 865630

Books

Bodily Communication
Michael Argyle 1988 (second edition) Routledge

A Sensory Curriculum for Very Special People
Flo Longhorn 1988 Souvenir Press

The Stimulation Guide
F.J. Dale 1990 Woodhead Faulkner

Touch: An Exploration
Norman Autton 1989 Darton Longman & Todd

Touching: The Human Significance of Skin
Ashley Montagu 1986 (third edition) Harper & Row

Visual Stimulation Videos

Cyberdelia (60 min)

Computer graphics transferred to video, with a soundtrack of Techno music. The video is divided into sections with different visual effects, some in black and white and others in brilliant colours. Some of the patterns change very rapidly and may not be suitable for people who have epilepsy, but others are slower. Produced by Prism Leisure; order from video stockists (especially HMV and W.H.Smith).

Fantasia (115 min)

Popular animated film with a soundtrack of classical music. Not as visually stimulating as one would like (try watching in a dark room and adjust colour and brightness controls to get the best effect) but the great thing about Fantasia is that the action is linked to the music. Produced by the Walt Disney Company; hire from video shops.

The Fractal Experience (30 min)

Computer graphics transferred to video, with a soundtrack of New Age music. Relaxing patterns in beautiful colours. Produced by Prism Leisure; order from video stockists (especially HMV and W.H.Smith).

Merak (50 min)

A space fantasy in light and sound. The video is in three sections: a spaceship journey; kaleidoscope patterns with gentle music and sounds; brightly coloured, fast moving patterns with lively music. Available from:
The Music Suite, Cenarth, Newcastle Emlyn, Dyfed SA38 9JN
Tel: 0239 710594.

Music and Sounds

Many of the educational and specialist catalogues include musical instruments; these companies specialize in them, especially instruments from different cultures:

Acorn Percussion
Unit 34, Abbey Business Centre, Ingate Place, London SW8 3NS
Tel: 071 720 2243   Fax: 071 627 3020

Knock on Wood
Arch X, Granary Wharf, The Canal Basin, Leeds LS1 4BR
Tel: 0532 429146

London Music Shop
Bedwas House Industrial Estate, Bedwas, Newport, Gwent NP1 8XQ
Tel: 0222 865775   Fax: 0222 851056

Natural sound Recordings

Three 'Earthsounds' cassettes — beach, woodland and stream — are available from:
Winslow Press
Telford Road, Bicester OX6 0TS
Tel: 0800 243755   Fax: 0869 320040

Cassettes of natural sounds, including tapes made to your own specification (chalk downland or Yorkshire moors, for instance) are available from:
Ken Jackson, 'Sounds Natural', Upper End, Fulbrook, Oxford OX8 4BX.

Music Tapes

A wide selection of musical styles should be available in good high-street record shops. Knock on Wood (see above) supply a range of music from around the world. Past Times (phone 0993 779339 for a copy of their catalogue or details of shops) often have tapes of Tudor music, old English country dances, etc.

My music collection includes:

Music from the Andes	East meets East (Japanese flute and sitar)
Music of Bali	Gipsy Kings
Steel band	Gamelin music
Missa Luba (mass sung in Congolese)	Music of the Tudor Age
Irish folk music	Brass band
Gregorian chant	Louis Jordan — Jump Jive
Dave Brubeck (jazz)	Bix Beiderbecke (jazz)
Dudley Moore (piano)	Evelyn Glennie (percussion)
Kenny Gee (saxaphone)	James Galway (flute)
John Williams (guitar)	Mike Oldfield
Jean Michel Jarre	Vangelis — music from the 'Chariots of
Kraftwerk — 'Autobahn'	Fire' soundtrack
Sinead O'Connor	Sade
Clannad	Enya
Capercaillie	

plus a range of classical and operatic music.

Soundbeam

Movement within the invisible Soundbeam 'plays' electronic keyboards. The beam can also be linked to multisensory effects and a vibrating board. A video is available, which shows Soundbeam in use in various settings. Demonstrations and training sessions are available. A supplement in 'Information Exchange' (see chapter 10) shares the latest information on developments and new applications.

The Soundbeam Project
463 Earlham Road, Norwich, Norfolk NR4 7HL
Tel: 0603 507788   Fax: 0603 507877

Musical Mat and Musical Presents

The Touch'n'Play Music Buttons required for these designs are available from:
The Craft Depot
1 Canvin Court, Somerton Business Park, Somerton, Somerset TA11 6SB
Tel/Fax: 0458 74727

Training

Contact the National Music and Disability Information Service, Foxhole, Dartington, Totnes, Devon TQ9 6EB, Tel: 0803 866701

Books

Some of these books are primarily about children with disabilities but contain some useful material for people working in adult services:

Music for the Handicapped child
Juliette Alvin 1965 Oxford University Press

Music for Mentally Handicapped People
Miriam Wood 1983 Souvenir Press

Music Therapy for the Autistic Child
Juliette Alvin 1978 Oxford University Press

Therapy in Music for Handicapped Children
Paul Nordoff and Clive Robbins 1985 Victor Gollancz

They Can Make Music
Philip Bailey 1973 Oxford University Press

Aromatherapy

Essential oils and other aromatherapy products are available from:

Shirley Price Aromatherapy
Upper Bond Street, Hinckley, Leics LE10 1RD
Tel: 0455 615466   Fax: 0455 615054

The Tisserand Institute
65 Church Road, Hove, Sussex BN3 2BD
Tel: 0273 206640/772479

Training

Courses are organized by:

Shirley Price Aromatherapy (see above) — general courses.
Hands On Training — courses on aromatherapy for people with learning disabilities.
9 Poplar Road, Kings Heath, Birmingham B14 7AA
Tel: 021 444 8057

Video

A video is available which gives a good introduction to aromatherapy — what essential oils are, how to mix and blend them, simple massage techniques. It is called 'Aromatherapy and massage' (60 min) and is available from video stockists or from Shirley Price Aromatherapy (see above).

Books

Aromatherapy
Micheline Arcier 1990 Hamlyn

Aromatherapy and Massage for People with Learning Difficulties
Helen Sanderson and Jane Harrison with Shirley Price 1991 Hands on Publishing (9 Poplar Road, Kings Heath, Birmingham B14 7AA).

Aromatherapy Workbook
Marcel Lavabre 1990 Healing Arts Press

The Book of Massage
Lucinda Lidell 1984 Ebury

The Massage Book
George Downing 1972 Penguin

Practical Aromatherapy
Shirley Price 1987 Thorsons

Movement

Training

Courses are organized by:

EXTEND
22 Maltings Drive, Wheathampstead, Herts AL4 8QJ
Tel: 0582 832760

EXTEND organizes recreational music and movement classes for elderly and disabled people. They provide training and tutors to work with groups.

Cyndi and George Hill, 1 The Vale, Parkfield, Nr. Pucklechurch BS17 3NW
Organize training courses using Veronica Sherborne's methods.

Video

Building Bridges (28 min)
This video shows movement classes for young people and adults with learning disabilities. The activities are presented as enjoyable games and encourage the participants to build relationships and develop self image. Available on hire or sale from:
Concord Video and Film Council
201 Felixstowe Road, Ipswich IP3 9BJ
Tel: 0473 726012

Books and Packs

Activity Programmes for Body Awareness, Contact and Communication
Marianne and Chris Knill LDA 1986
Available from: LDA, Duke Street, Wisbech PE13 2AE; Tel: 0945 63441 or Winslow Press, Telford Road, Bicester OX6 0TS; Tel: 0800 243755

Body and Voice
Carrie Lennard (ed.) LDA 1987
Available from LDA or Winslow Press (see above).
(Intended for use with children, but many of the songs are suitable for adults.)

Creative Movement and Dance in Groupwork
Helen Payne 1990 Winslow Press (see above)

Developmental Movement for Children
Veronica Sherborne Cambridge University Press 1990
(This book is about her work with children but the underlying principles apply equally well to adults.)

No Handicap to Dance
Gina Levete 1982 Souvenir Press

Sensory-Motor Integration Activities
Barbara Fink
Available from Winslow Press (see above).

Yoga

YOU & ME

This is a yoga system, devised by Maria Gunstone, for people with learning disabilities. The system involves the therapeutic use of colour, sound and whole body movement and many of the body postures are suitable for people with profound disabilities.

A handbook, teaching pack, and a report and video entitled 'Yoga therapy and special education in India' are all available from:

Maria Gunstone, YOU & ME
The Cottage, Burton-in-Kendal, Carnforth LA6 1ND
Tel: 0524 782103

Training

Courses in the YOU & ME system of yoga are organized by Maria Gunstone (see above). Information on other training courses is available from:

The British Wheel of Yoga
1 Hamilton Place, Boston Road, Sleaford NG32 7ES

Yoga for Health Foundation
Ickwell Bury, Northill, Biggleswade SG18 9EF

Books

Yoga for Handicapped People
Barbara Brosnan 1982 Souvenir Press

Yoga for the Disabled
Howard Kent 1985 Thorsons

Multisensory Environments (chapter 5)

The following companies supply equipment for multisensory environments, most also offer a design service:

Environmental Electrical Services (CAVE)
Manywells House, Manywells Industrial Estate, Cullingworth, Bradford BD13 5DX
Tel: 0535 274068

Grayhirst Training and Consultancy
7 Elsemere Road, Morecambe LA4 5LF
Tel: 0524 426395
and
29 Elizabeth Road, Sutton Coldfield B73 5AR
Tel: 021 355 2089

Kirton Litework
Unit 2, Woodgate Park, White Lund Industrial Estate, Morecambe LA3 3PS
Tel: 0524 844808

Messenger & Clark
Pious Drive, Upwell, Wisbech PE14 9AN
Tel: 0945 773627 or 0902 895991

Mike Ayres Design
Unit 8, Shepherds Grove, Stanton, Bury St Edmunds, Suffolk IP31 2AR
Tel: 0359 251551   Fax: 0359 251707

Rompa
Goyt Side Road, Chesterfield S40 2PH
Tel: 0246 211777

Sense-Ability
Unit 1, Woodgate Park, White Lund Industrial Estate, Morecambe LA3 3PS
Tel: 0524 846946

Spacekraft
Crowgill House, Rosse Street, Shipley BD18 3SW
Tel: 0274 581966

TFH
76 Barracks Road, Sandy Lane Industrial Estate, Stourport-on-Severn DY13 9QB
Tel: 0299 827820

These companies supply individual items which may be useful:

Flying Objects (pale coloured parachutes, for creating environments)
The Basement, 29 Meridan Place, Bristol, Avon BS8 1JL
Tel/Fax: 0272 525262

Innovations (Mail Order) Ltd (rope lights)
Euroway Business Park, Swindon SN5 8SN
Tel: 0793 513946

International Buyers Guide (rope lights, battery-powered Christmas-tree lights)
Euroway Business Park, Swindon SN5 8SN
Tel: 0793 513946

Training

Courses on the use of multisensory rooms are organized by:

Grayhirst Training & Consultancy (see above)
RNIB — MVHI Training Service,
c/o RNIB, 224-228 Great Portland Street,
London W1N 6AA
Tel: 071 388 1266

Rompa (see above).

Videos

Snoezelen (18 min)
Illustrates the use of Snoezelen in special education, leisure and elderly care. More useful as an aid for fundraising, or to show the concept of Snoezelen, than as a training tool for staff. Available from Rompa (see above).

The White Tower (10 min)
Shows how to use a selection of equipment which might be found in a multisensory environment. Available from TFH (see above).

Books

Snoezelen: another world, Jan Hulsegge and Ad Verheul 1987 Rompa (see above)

Relaxation Music

Mike Ayres & Co. and Rompa supply tapes of relaxation music. For a more comprehensive selection, contact:

New Age Experience
27 Market Place, Penzance TR18 6HD
Tel: 0736 50055

New World Cassettes
Paradise Farm, Westhall, Halesworth, Suffolk IP19 8RH
Tel: 050 279 279   Fax: 050 279 886.

Theme Work

Galaxies and Seaside are available from:

Resources for Learning Difficulties
The Consortium, Jack Tizard School, Finlay Street, London SW6 6HB
Tel: 071 736 8877

Sensory Gardens

For advice on designing and constructing sensory gardens, contact:

Horticultural Therapy
Goulds Ground, Vallis Way, Frome, Somerset BA11 3DW
Tel: 0373 64782

RNIB
Leisure Department, RNIB, 224-228 Great Portland Street, London W1N 6AA
Tel: 071-388 1266

Creating (chapter 5)

Most of the educational catalogues include art and craft materials; these are also available from:

Dryad Specialist Crafts
PO Box 247, Leicester LE1 9QS
Tel: 0533 510405   Fax: 0533 515015

Books

Arts and Disabled People: The Attenborough Report
Carnegie UK Trust 1985

Creative and Mental Growth
Viktor Lowenfeld and W. Lambert Brittain 1982 Macmillan

Creative Arts and Mental Disability
Stanley S. Segal (ed.) 1990 AB Academic Publishers

The Creative Tree: Active Participation in the Arts for People who are Disadvantaged
Gina Levete (ed.) 1987 Michael Russell

Using the Creative Arts in Therapy
Bernie Warren (ed.) 1984 Croom Helm

Puppets

Suppliers include:

Ann Johnson
38 Gledhow Wood Grove, Leeds LS8 1NZ
Tel: 0532 667177
  Range of multi-ethnic hand puppets.

Dormouse Designs
The Old Drapery, Faith Avenue, Quarriers Village, By Bridge of Weir, Renfrewshire PA11 3SX
Tel: 0505 690435
  Large black and white sheep puppet which 'baas' when its head is raised.

Montoys
28 Woodcroft Avenue, Stanmore, Middx HA7 3PS
Tel: 081 954 5162
  Range of realistic animal glove puppets.

Books

The Knowhow Book of Puppets: a Simple Guide to Making and Working Puppets
Violet Philpott and Mary Jean McNeil 1975 Usborne

Puppetry for Mentally Handicapped People
Caroline Astell-Burt 1981 Souvenir Press

Games (chapter 8)

Suppliers

Karum's Karom Board Workshop
Annan Farm, Easons Green, East Sussex TN22 5RE
Tel: 0825 840574

New Games UK (flexible frisbees)
Stewart Abel, 28 Kendal Court, Shoot Up Hill, London NW2 3PD

Rink Products
13 Victoria Road North, Leicester LE4 5EX
Tel: 0533 666382

Sportime
Cemetery Lane, Carlton, Wakefield WF3 3QT
Tel: 0532 824494   Fax: 0532 824706

Boccia

Sets of Boccia balls are supplied by:

Newton Products
Meadway Works, Garretts Green Lane, Birmingham B33 0SQ
Tel: 021 783 6081

For further information about the sport, contact:

The National Boccia Association
11 Churchill Park, Colwick, Nottingham NG4 2HE

Meldreth Series Games

Two publications are available, giving details of the equipment and rules:

The Meldreth Series: Principle and Practice
Len Reed 1989
    Available from The Spastics Society, Meldreth Manor School, Meldreth, Royston, Herts.

The Meldreth Series: Old Games with a New Look for Severely Disabled People
Len Reed 1990
    Available as above.

A video, *Meldreth games* (32 min), is available from:

Cerebral Palsy Sport
11 Churchill Park, Colwick, Nottingham NG4 2HE
Tel: 0602 401202

    Training courses on the Meldreth games are organized by Pro-Motion (see chapter 10).

Adapted Games

Practical Innovations for Nine Adapted Activities, Games and Sports
Richard Smith and Doug Williamson (eds) 1992
    This practical manual is available from:
    Adapted Physical Activities Unit
    Department of Primary Education, Nottingham Polytechnic, Clifton Site, Nottingham NG11 8NS.

Co-operative Games

Training courses are organized by New Games UK, who also supply books and other materials. For information on the organization, contact:
PO Box 542, London NW2 3PQ.
For orders, contact:
Stewart Abel, 28 Kendal Court, Shoot Up Hill, London NW2 3PD.

Video

Let's Co-operate (20 min)
  Shows children playing a wide variety of co-operative games, several using a parachute. Games are suitable for adults. Available from: Mildred Masheder, 75 Belsize Lane, London NW3 5AU; Tel: 071 435 2182

Books

Games Games Games
Rachel Dewar, Kate Palser and Martin Notley 1989 The Woodcraft Folk

Gamesters' Handbook Two
Donna Brandes 1982 Hutchinson

Let's Co-operate
Mildred Masheder 1989 Peace Education Project
  Available from Play for Life (31B Ipswich Road, Norwich NR2 2LN).

The New Games Book
Andrew Fluegelman (ed.) 1976 Headlands Press
  Available from New Games UK (see above).

More New Games
Andrew Fluegelman 1981 Dolphin Books
  Available from New Games UK (see above)

Playfair: Everybody's Guide to Noncompetitive Play
Matt Weinstein and Joel Goodman 1980 Impact Publishers
  Available from New Games UK (see above)

Winners All: Co-operative Games for All Ages
Pax Christi 1980
  Available from Play for Life (see above)

Parachute Games

Parachutes are supplied by:

Flying Objects
The Basement, 29 Meridan Place, Bristol, Avon BS8 1JL
Tel/Fax: 0272 525262
  The parachutes are in plain, pale colours and are sold as part of a kit consisting of a 5 m diameter parachute plus two books and a video by Mildred Masheder (see above).

Sportime
Cemetery Lane, Carlton, Wakefield WF3 3QT
Tel: 0532 824494   Fax: 0532 824706
Supply bright multicoloured parachutes.

Kites

A few kites are available from Mike Ayres & Co. and Rompa. For a wider range, and the materials for making kites, contact:

Brookite
Brightley Mill, Okehampton, Devon EX20 1RR
Tel: 0837 53315   Fax: 0837 53223

Books

25 Kites That Fly
Leslie L. Hunt 1971 Dover Publications

Easy-to-Make Decorative Kites
Alan and Gill Bridgewater 1985 Constable

How to Make and Fly Kites
Eve Barwell and Conrad Bailey 1972 Studio Vista

The Penguin Book of Kites
David Pelham 1976 Penguin

Cycles

The following companies supply a range of cycles:

Howie Cycles
113 Main Street, Auchinleck, Strathclyde KA18 2AF
Tel: 0290 25910

Neatwork
PO Box 2, Coldstream, Berwickshire TD12 4NN
Tel: 0890 883456   Fax: 0890 882709

WRK
Ashfield House, School Road, St John's Fen End, Nr Wisbech PE14 7SJ
Tel: 0945 880014   Fax: 0945 880910

Booklist — General

There are some books which inspire because of the attitude and philosophy of the author:

The Other Side of Profound Handicap
Pat Brudenell 1986 Macmillan

Her approach to and consideration for the people she works with are combined with practical down-to-earth suggestions and ideas.

Play is a Feeling
Brenda Crowe 1983 Unwin
An exploration of childhood and those first experiences of sensation, movement, language and surroundings which are an essential part of our development. A reminder of our needs and feelings and the difficulties we faced when trying to explain to powerful adults what was important to us.

Are You Blind? Promotion of the Development of Children who are Especially Developmentally Threatened
Lilli Neilson1990

Educational Approaches for Visually Impaired Children
Lilli Neilson 1992

Space and Self
Lilli Neilson 1992
All published by SIKON and available from RNIB (224 Great Portland Street, London W1N 6AA).
Her unique insights and views on handling and educating children with visual impairments and other disabilities challenge the beliefs held by many professionals in this country, especially teachers. Much of her writing is relevant to adults with multiple disabilities.

Other useful books, for background reading or sources of new ideas:

Innovations in Leisure and Recreation for People with a Mental Handicap
Roy McConkey and Patrick McGinley 1990 Lisieux Hall

Leisure Resource Pack
Mencap PRMH Project 1991
Series of booklets and a videotape providing information on leisure for children and adults with profound and multiple disabilities. The PRMH Project has now been renamed the Mencap PIMD Section.
Available from Mencap PIMD Section, Piper Hill School, 200 Yew Tree Lane, Northenden, Manchester M23 0FF; Tel: 061 998 4161.

Persons with Profound Disabilities: Issues and Practices
Freda Brown and Donna H. Lehr 1989 Paul H. Brookes

Profound Retardation and Multiple Impairment
Vol 1 Development and Learning
Vol. 2 Education and therapy
James Hogg and Judy Sebba 1986 Croom Helm
Vol 3 Medical and Physical Care and Management
James Hogg, Judy Sebba and Loretto Lambe 1990 Chapman and Hall

Index